OXFORD
G N V Q

Restricted
Loan

Intermediate

HEALTH & SOCIAL CARE

This ... to be returned on or before ... date stamped below

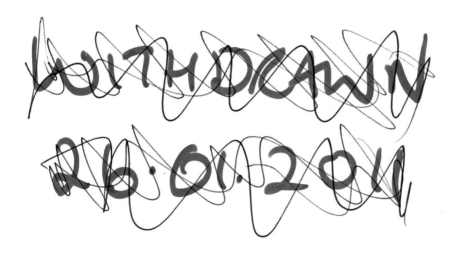

WITHDRAWN

26.01.2011

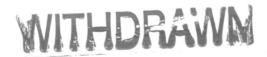

WITHDRAWN

Christine Barratt

Buckinghamshire College Group
Wycombe Campus

Oxford University Press

Oxford University Press, Walton Street, Oxford OX2 6DP

Oxford New York
Athens Auckland Bangkok Bombay
Calcutta Cape Town Dar es Salaam Delhi
Florence Hong Kong Istanbul Karachi
Kuala Lumpur Madras Madrid Melbourne
Mexico City Nairobi Paris Singapore
Taipei Tokyo Toronto
and associated companies in
Berlin Ibadan

Oxford is a trade mark of Oxford University Press

First published 1996

ISBN 0 19 832796 X

Typesetting by Pentacor PLC

Illustration by Hilary Earl, David Huggins, Gordon Lawson, Peter Marsh,
Oxford Illustrators, Geo Parkin, Julie Tolliday and Lynn Williams.

Printed in Spain by Gráficas Estella, S.A.

*The publisher would like to thank the following for their kind permission to
reproduce the following photographs:*

Ace Photo Agency **page 86 bl** Michael Bluestone, **page 114 al** Lesley
Howling; Anthony Blake Photo Library/Andrew Sydenham **page 24 bc**; A-Z
Botanical **page 56 bl** Jiri Loun, **page 56 bcl** W. Broadhurst, **page 56 bcr**
Steven Owens, **page 56 br** F. Merlet; Collections **page 79 cl & cr** Anthea
Sieveking; Courtesy Coopers Healthcare Plc **page 220** all photos except top
centre; Courtesy Dolphin Lifts **page 220** top centre; Food Features **page 24
bl & br**; Format **page 21 al** Maggie Murray, **page 79 bl** Jacky Chapman
page 85 cl Judy Harrison, **page 99 cr** Paula Solloway, **page 114 ar** Ulrike
Preuss, **page 175 a** Maggie Murray; Sally Greenhill **page 39 cl**, **79 br**, **175
b**; Richard Greenhill **page 195 bl**; Sally & Richard Greenhill **page 114 bl &
115 al**: Health Education Authority **page 40 al**; Courtesy Rexam Medical
Packaging **page 29 br**; RNIB **page 146 bc** Tony Sleep, **page 146 br** Sally
Lancaster, **page 175 c** Sally Lancaster; Stockfile/Steven Behr **page 54 cl**;
TRIP **page 86 cl** J. Highet, **page 86 cr** J. Wakelin, **page 86 br** P. Rauter,
page 99 cl M. Lee, **page 114 br** H. Rogers

Key   a - above; **b** - below; **l** - left; **r** - right; **c** - centre.

Cover photo - Collections/Anthea Sieveking

*The publisher would like to thank the staff and students of Abingdon College
for trialling some of the text.*

Contents

		Page
Acknowledgements		
Introduction		**5**
Core Skills Preface		**13**
1 Application of Number		13
2 Information technology		14
3 Communication		16
Unit 1	**Promoting health and well-being**	**18**
Element 1.1	Investigate personal health	19
Element 1.2	Present advice on health and well-being to others	36
Element 1.3	Reduce risk of injury and deal with emergencies	51
Unit 2	**Influences on health and well-being**	**73**
Element 2.1	Explore the development of individuals and how they manage change	74
Element 2.2	Explore the nature of inter-personal relationships and their influence on health and well-being	97
Element 2.3	Explore the interactions of individuals within society and how they may influence health and well-being	113
Unit 3	**Health and Social care services**	**128**
Element 3.1	Investigate the provision of health and social care services	129
Element 3.2	Describe how the needs of different clients are met by health and social services	145
Element 3.3	Investigate jobs in health and social care	159
Unit 4	**Communication and interpersonal relationships**	**172**
Element 4.1	Develop communication skills	173
Element 4.2	Explore how inter-personal relationships may be affected by discriminatory behaviour	193
Element 4.3	Investigate aspects of working with clients in health and social care	210
Index		**232**
Answers		**232**

Acknowledgements

I am indebted to a number of valued colleagues for their expert advice and inspiration. Initial encouragement came from Mary Dunn of Hampshire County Council's Education Department, Sylvia Law of Farnborough College of Technology, and Angela Brice from Itchen College.

Prue Amner, of Highbury College of Technology, and George Newton, from Bridgemary School, have provided the specialist Information Technology and Application of Number content.

Julia Priestley, of the Gosport Guidance and Careers Service, and members of Fareham and Gosport Magistrates' bench have kindly checked all the sections falling within their professional spheres.

Kim Bridgen and Karen Matthews have tussled with my handwriting to type the manuscript. My family has provided continual support and encouragement, and I would like to dedicate this book to Sarah, our daughter.

It has been my good fortune to work with these people and others who have helped in different ways.

Christine Barratt

1996

Introduction

About the GNVQ

The General National Vocational Qualification in Health and Social Care offers you a wide background knowledge of work in this occupational field. Gaining a certificate for the Intermediate level will equip you to

1 apply for a job

2 progress to further study, such as Advanced level GNVQ or GCE A level subjects, and then into higher education at college or university

3 work towards a National Vocational Qualification (NVQ). The two especially relevant NVQs are in Care, and Child Care and Education.

A wider range of career opportunities is described in Unit 3 Element 3, which may help you to decide what you will do after you have completed your Intermediate level award.

To gain an Intermediate GNVQ you will have to complete nine units:

- four **mandatory** units
- three **core skills** units
- two **optional** units.

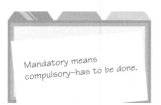

Mandatory means compulsory–has to be done.

The mandatory and core skills units are covered in this book. The optional units are not included. They vary according to which of the three awarding bodies – BTEC, the City and Guilds of London Institute, or the RSA Examinations Board – designs them. You will select two from several optional units offered by the awarding body with whom you are registered by your school or college. Your teacher or lecturer will explain the choices to you and guide you through them.

The mandatory units

Each of the four **mandatory units** is made up of three **elements**. In some units the first element gives the foundation knowledge you need to proceed to the following elements.

Each element has

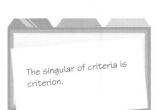

The singular of criteria is criterion.

- several **performance criteria.** These are called **pcs** for short. They state what you have to do
- a **range** which describes the details you have to cover
- **evidence indicators** which outline the sort of evidence you need to produce.

The structure of the four mandatory units of the Intermediate GNVQ in Health and Social Care

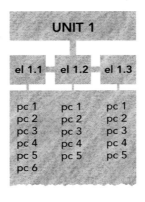

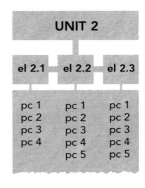

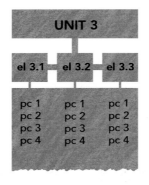

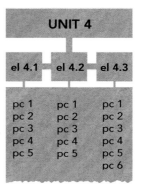

In order to gain a full **level**, all four units have to be achieved, but you can have individual units certificated. It is not possible to have a certificate for separate elements.

Assessment

Assessment involves judgement and grading. The four mandatory units are judged and graded by

- **internal** assessment by your school or college
- **external** assessment by your awarding body.

You have to collect evidence of your ability and knowledge in a **portfolio**, which needs to cover the performance criteria and range to show the depth of your knowledge. Your portfolio will be internally assessed in your school or college, and the assessment confirmed by the representative of the awarding body, who is called an **external verifier**.

External assessment includes **multiple choice tests** for Units 1, 2 and 3. These are set by the awarding bodies.

It is possible to gain a **pass**, **merit** or **distinction**. To achieve a pass you must have completed your portfolio and also been successful in the multiple choice test. Teaching staff will explain to you how merits and distinctions can be achieved.

Core skills

As well as understanding health and social care, you also have to show knowledge of additional general skills. These are known as **core skills**, and are

- Application of Number
- Information Technology
- Communication.

They themselves have units, each with their own elements, performance criteria and range. You will be examining aspects of their use in health and social care; the activities suggested in the text offer simple opportunities for demonstrating your competence at a basic standard. Aspects which are not covered in the text are explained in the Core Skills Preface on page 13.

The core skills are designed on five **levels** – this book concentrates on level 2. If you are particularly skilled in one or all of the core skills, it is possible for you to achieve a higher level while completing your Intermediate programme. For this you will need guidance from your teaching staff.

About this book

This book aims to lead you through the knowledge requirements laid down in the four mandatory units, at the same time helping you to put together evidence for your portfolio through activities, case studies and questions in the tasks.

The book is in four sections and each section covers one unit. Each section has an introduction to the unit content, followed by subsections on each of the three elements in that unit. Each element follows the pattern of

- knowledge and activities
- case studies
- multiple choice questions
- summary of evidence opportunities and their relationship to the performance criteria
- summary of element range and personal evidence tracking record.

Knowledge and activities

Each element is introduced with a list of its performance criteria. Then each performance criterion is taken in turn, with activities which allow you to gather evidence of your knowledge and understanding. This evidence will need to be placed in your portfolio with a reference number so that it can be found easily.

You will be given ideas for presenting the suggested evidence using techniques from the core skills range, but you may need specialist help from your teacher or lecturer in achieving the core skills' own performance criteria. Aspects of all three – Application of Number, Information Technology and Communication – that are important for you to understand before you begin are outlined in the Core Skills Preface (page 13).

Where you see the symbol ◀▶ this indicates **extension opportunities**. These give you the chance to extend your understanding and knowledge of a particular area. Take advantage of them if you are aiming for a merit or distinction grade; it will show that you are prepared to work independently. They will also give you ideas for developing other activities further if you wish to. The same symbol will also be used to indicate **core skills opportunities**.

Case studies

The case studies are based on the following four fictitious organisations:

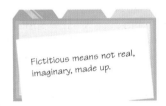

Fictitious means not real, imaginary, made up.

1 Netherfield Community Care team

2 Hill Hall, a school for children and young adults with profound learning difficulties

3 The Thatched Cottage residential care home

4 Down Way School

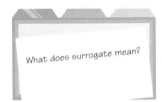

What does surrogate mean?

These four establishments, described in detail on page 9, will provide you with surrogate placements if you are not able to visit care organisations on your course of study. The scenarios described are intended to be as realistic as possible, all examples being drawn from actual care work experiences.

Multiple choice questions

These are intended to make you familiar with the sort of question in the unit tests, while giving you the opportunity to gather some **supplementary evidence**, that is, small items of extra evidence to cover the element range. (Remember that the multiple choice unit tests are only for mandatory units 1, 2 and 3.)

Summary of information, evidence opportunities and tracking systems

At the end of each element is a table summarising its range. This will enable you to see at a glance where the text has given you the opportunity to produce evidence. On a photocopy you will be able to tick off your evidence as the range is covered, and see where you need to do further work. There is space too for cross-referencing your evidence, which will help you with the organisation of your portfolio.

The GNVQ system encourages students **to take responsibility for their own learning**. The activities suggested in the book offer you the opportunity to achieve minimum coverage of the Health and Social Care performance criteria, and core skills techniques as already described. You may choose to expand them. Remember that books like this one are not your only resources. Television, newspapers, radio, films, and magazines regularly discuss the matters of human interest on which your GNVQ units focus.

Look at your own and your friends' and family's life experiences. Bring these to bear in your evidence, which will become more lively and realistic, up to date and thoughtful. You must, of course, make sure that any facts you choose to present are from an accurate and reliable source, and that if the people involved are friends or clients you get their permission to use their experiences in this way.

Confidentiality is a key issue in the field of health and social care. It is covered specifically in Unit 4 Element 3, but is worth a mention here in the context of case studies and work experience. Every student must be aware of the need for confidentiality in all aspects of caring, including any written work which may follow visits outside the school or college. This will have to be discussed with your teacher or lecturer, and the supervisor in any place of work.

You will find **'fact file-cards'** scattered throughout the book. These are intended to clarify words and phrases used in the text. You might like to keep a glossary or dictionary of the most useful; many will help to expand your professional language.

The Case Study Establishments

Netherfield Community Care

Mikhail

Netherfield is a sprawling urban area. It has expanded from an industrial heartland to encompass several surrounding villages. The community is mixed, ranging from an ageing local population through a strong Polish community to young people attracted to small, affordable high rise flats. Some areas of the town are depressed.

A community team works in this environment. The Community Care Act has increased their responsibilities considerably. There have always been clients who very much preferred to stay independent in their own homes despite requiring care, but now several hostels for people with mental health problems have opened. The Netherfield community team is responding by taking on trained staff able to meet this new need.

The members of the community care team feel that community care work is very rewarding,

Debbie

demanding and stimulating, and are keen to encourage people to consider it as a career. With this in mind they welcome students from Netherfield College on work placement, both those straight from school and mature students.

The health care worker who organises the work experience of students is Mikhail, a young Polish national. He is an idealist, but his training has made his attitude more realistic without quashing his dreams.

He transmits his enthusiasm for community care to the students in his care. He is dedicated to improving the quality of life for all clients while naturally relating well to the Polish community. His English is almost perfect.

Debbie is a student who loves the variety given by community care. She is distressed by the financial restraints affecting services, and is resisting Mikhail's attempts to encourage her to accept the situation without causing a fuss.

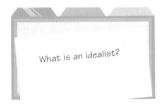

What is an idealist?

Hill Hall

Hill Hall is a school catering for children from 3 to 19 years of age from a wide surrounding area, who arrive by bus, taxi, and private transport each day. All the children have severe learning difficulties, and require constant care alongside their education. The school aims to provide the opportunity for all pupils to meet their potential. Most will never be able to integrate into society. Some die while they are still children. Others succeed against all odds. Staff are somewhat dissatisfied. The school is very expensive to maintain and it is rumoured that it will close in five years time.

The resources are excellent – it has a hydrotherapy bath, and a Schnoozlen room in which children can listen to gentle music and experience a variety of lighting effects and different touch and smell sensations in complete safety. The dedicated staff are skilled in meeting all the pupils' needs, including physiotherapy and special diets.

The school is set in the centre of a city and welcomes students from the local college for work experience, although it is aware that the work makes special demands. The severity of the children's disabilities can be difficult for some carers to come to terms with.

Molly is a dedicated senior care worker, who has worked in the school team for many years. She is devoted to the children, and is committed to the

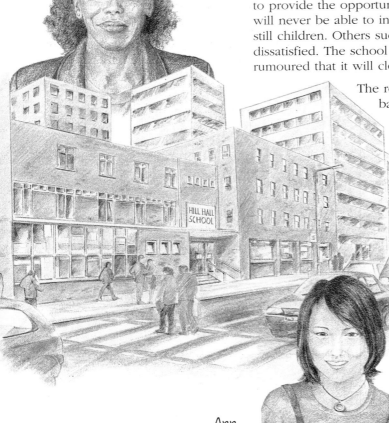

Molly

Ann

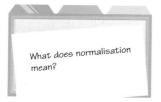

What does normalisation mean?

normalisation process. She is the person to whom placement students naturally turn, as she is approachable and sympathetic.

The student at present on placement at Hill Hall is Ann, who is very new to this type of work and finding it hard to come to grips with the severity of the children's disabilities. She is quiet and does not share her anxieties easily. Her first inclination is to go off sick when things alarm her, but she is trying to overcome this. She sleeps badly, as she worries about her attitude and wonders if she has chosen the wrong course.

The Thatched Cottage

The Thatched Cottage is a residential home by the sea. It has 23 residents, mostly elderly. Some have been transferred from a local hospital for people with moderate learning disabilities which has recently closed down.

Some residents are able bodied, while others are handicapped by a variety of complaints ranging from arthritis to chronic bronchitis. Some are confused, others are alert. Public transport is limited. There is a pub, a post office and a few shops nearby with a tea room up the road. The nearest churches are about a mile away. The ground falls steeply to the sea outside the house. The gardens are big enough to hold summer fetes and other activities, but not flat enough for residents with mobility problems to stroll far.

Dora

Mark

In addition to its usual staff, The Thatched Cottage welcomes college and secondary school pupils on work experience, and has other staff on employment training.

Dora is the senior care assistant in The Thatched Cottage. She has ten years' experience, and has recently been put in charge of managing new care assistants and all those working on a temporary or short-term basis in the home. She is therefore the line manager of students on placement.

You will be following the progress of Mark, a student from the local college. He is not sure what he wants to do after completing his course, but enjoys working with the residents as it gives him a wide range of caring experience. He knows that it will come in useful, and will also strengthen his letters of application for work.

A line manager is someone responsible for certain other workers, from whom they can seek guidance and advice.

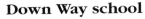

Isabel

Jalwinder

Down Way school

Down Way School is a rural primary school. It was built in Edwardian times and many of the children's parents attended in their childhood. The number of pupils has fallen recently. Now that there is room for it, the school has opened a small nursery/playgroup in one of its biggest classrooms. A new housing estate is being developed nearby, and the children living there will attend Down Way next September.

There are at present 106 children, the youngest being two and a half and the oldest eleven. When they leave the older children move on to the local comprehensive school about a mile away. Young people who used to attend the school return to Down Way for work experience, and college students also visit on a placement basis for vocational courses.

Isabel is a non-teaching assistant at the school. She began helping voluntarily as a mother when her children were small, and later gained a part-time post; she now works full time. She knows a great deal about the school, and has moved about into different classes as the school has changed. She is very much looking forward to seeing numbers grow, and has helped a great deal with the development of the nursery, as she has had playgroup experience.

Jalwinder is a Punjabi health care student on placement at Down Way. She wants to run her own nursery school eventually. She is a cheerful, competent girl and finds her creative skills useful when working with the children.

Now read on. Enjoy your studies. In the end they will enable you to enter into a lifetime of stimulating and rewarding work in one of the caring professions.

Core Skills Preface

1 Application of Number

Elements

2.1 Collect and record data

2.2 Tackle problems

2.3 Interpret and present data

You will be offered opportunities to gather evidence for part of all three elements. In several cases you will be able to combine the evidence with that for Information Technology. You may be able to find further possibilities for combining the core skills for yourself.

However, you will need to read the performance criteria in order to complete them in detail. In particular, you will need to demonstrate your ability to work with shapes, spaces and measures. You will have to complete the fine details of some performance criteria through extra activities devised by you or your teacher or lecturer.

Element 2.1

You will be able to compile most of your evidence for this element by following the guidelines in the text. You may need help from teaching staff to interpret which of the techniques described in the element range have been covered.

Element 2.2

There are many evidence opportunities in the Health and Safety units, but they will need adding to for total coverage of the range.

Volume is not covered. You could devise an activity in which you measured the volume of a room – *depth* **x** *width* **x** *height* – in order to estimate its ventilation needs. In working out the volume of a cylinder, think about syringes, jugs and babies' bottles to make the exercise relevant to the care field.

Element 2.3

Most performance criteria are covered, but you will need additional opportunities to enable you to show your competence in making two-dimensional images of three-dimensional objects.

Where the term **probability** is used, it may also cover

- estimation
- levels of accuracy
- tolerance.

2 Information Technology (IT)

Elements

2.1 Prepare information

2.2 Process information

2.3 Present information

2.4 Evaluate the use of information technology

Evidence opportunities for the first three elements are offered through the activities in the text. The fourth element is not easy to cover in the same way, and some of the performance criteria cannot be completed until you have gained enough computer experience to analyse. For instance, you are asked in Element 2.4 to explain why information technology is useful in relation to particular tasks. For this you could consider how you have used a computer to improve your portfolio, and this will have to be done by looking back at your work.

The supplementary activities which follow will give you the chance to demonstrate your IT competence. There is also a short section on health and safety connected with computer use.

DON'T FORGET TO COME BACK TO THESE ACTIVITIES LATER.

IT ACTIVITY 1

[Element 2.4, pc 4]

While you are using the computer several errors or faults will occur. Some will be due to your own inexperience. Some will be unavoidable. Whichever they are, enter the event on a log sheet. Draw up two columns; What went wrong. How was it put right. Then, whenever you have a problem, note who corrected it or how you solved it yourself. By the end of the GNVQ programme you will then have evidence that you can deal with many problems.

IT ACTIVITY 2

[Element 2.4, pcs 1, 2, 3]

1 Consider some of the activities where you have used the computer to prepare work. Explain how useful you find it in terms of
  - speed
  - effort
  - ease of use
  - accuracy.
2 How have you improved? Have your attitudes changed?
3 What software did you use?

IT ACTIVITY 3

[Element 2.4 pcs 1, 3, 4]

While on work experience, or by interviewing an appropriate person, find out how an establishment uses or could use computers. Record
  - why computers are found to be useful
  - what they produce
  - how they help the organisation
  - what the benefits are.

Working safely

There are guidelines on minimum requirements for computer systems furniture which are as follows:

Display screen
- must have ability to be read with a stable picture and no flicker
- be able to adjust brightness, contrast, tilt and swivel easily
- must have no reflections

Keyboard
- must be separate from the screen and tiltable
- placed on a matt surface to avoid glare
- have easy to use layout
- easy to read labels
- sufficient desk space for hand and arm support

Desk
- must be large enough for flexible arrangement of equipment and papers
- must have low reflectance
- enough space for people to change position.

Lights
- must have appropriate contrast between screen and background
- no glare or reflections
- adjustable coverings for windows

Noise – not loud enough to distract or disturb speech

Chair
- must be adjustable, comfortable and allow freedom of movement
- must have access to a footrest if requested

Software
- should be easy to use and appropriate to user's needs and experience
- able to provide feedback on performance – performance checks without the workers' knowledge are illegal

Other matters – heat, humidity and radiation emissions must be at 'adequate levels'

Health risks – the main physical risks are
- musculo-skeletal problems such as repetitive strain injury (RSI)
- visual fatigue
- mental stress

These are minimised by good working environment, job design and posture.

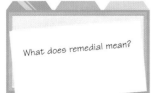

What does remedial mean?

IT ACTIVITY 4

[Element 2.4, pcs 4 and 5]

1   Make a checklist for inspecting a computer workstation or a computer room.

2   Carry out an inspection using your checklist.

3   Against each item on your checklist report the situation you found.

4   If necessary, at the end of your report make a list of remedial actions required to bring the workstation up to acceptable standards.

3 Communication

Elements

2.1 Take part in discussions

2.2 Produce written material

2.3 Use images

2.4 Read and respond to written materials

In the suggested activities you will not be given many specific references to make sure that you cover the communication core skills requirements as the opportunities will be too numerous. However, you may find it helpful to read the following points before you begin.

Discussions

Make sure that you take an active and useful part in discussions and that at least two group and two one-to-one discussions are assessed and recorded. One must be with people who know about the subject but who do not know you. Use discussions on several different subjects and for several different purposes. Use them to obtain information, give information and exchange your views with other people.

Written material

- Written information must be relevant, which means that it must fulfil the intended purpose.

- Handwriting must be easy to read.

- The contents need to be understandable and thorough.

- Pay attention to your spelling, punctuation and grammar.

- Present your work in as many different ways as possible – you will be given plenty of scope in the activities suggested in the text.

- Use a style which helps to make your meaning clear.

- Make it suitable for readers who know you and readers who may never meet you.

Images

- This means pictures, diagrams, maps, sketches – any information which is not solely in words.

- Design some of your own and use others from books.

- Make them suitable for their purpose.

- Select some for presentation in your written work.

- Think about using images to illustrate points in the discussions – photocopying, sheets or transparencies for overhead projection, posters and photographs.

- Record your use of images in explaining things to people who know you and people who do not know you.

- Use appropriate work from your Application of Number and IT core skills.

- Think about making videos to combine images with words.

Reading and responding to written material

- Activities will give you the chance to study text (which means words alone), and text combined with images (pictures, graphs, diagrams, etc.).

- Use many sources in addition to books – notices, tables, newspaper and magazine articles, etc.

- Confirm your understanding of the information by asking questions and reading more about it to make sure of its accuracy.

- Write about what you have found out.

- Talk about what you have found out.

  (The last two points will be covered in Elements 2.1 and 2.2).

- Use summaries, that is, brief accounts summing up the subject you have been studying.

Unit 4 is all about communication and will give you many chances to demonstrate your skills. Remember that you will also be communicating when you talk about Application of Number to members of your teaching staff. Numbers are as important as words in communication..

Your IT work will give you further opportunities to display information by using a computer – another type of communication.

You will see that, as you get used to the idea of combining the core skills, you will have ample opportunity to demonstrate your ability to communicate. Remember to keep a log so that your competence can be recorded and assessed properly.

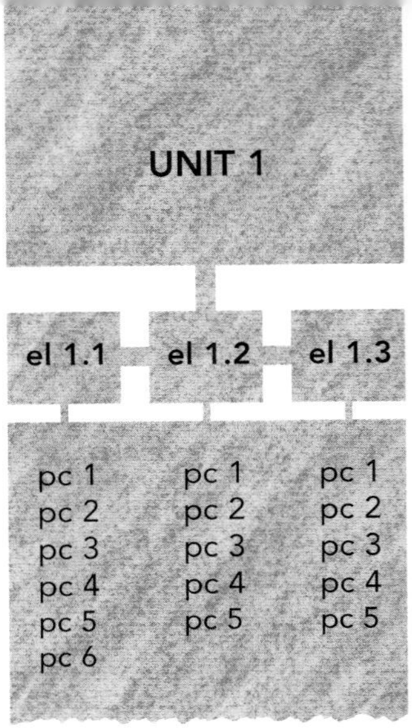

Unit

one

UNIT 1		
el 1.1	el 1.2	el 1.3
pc 1	pc 1	pc 1
pc 2	pc 2	pc 2
pc 3	pc 3	pc 3
pc 4	pc 4	pc 4
pc 5	pc 5	pc 5
pc 6		

Promoting Health and Well-Being

Elements

1.1 Investigate personal health

1.2 Present advice on health and well-being to others

1.3 Reduce risk of injury and deal with emergencies

This unit aims to help you to understand personal health and well-being, both your own, and that of the people with whom you may be working. You will be learning how to keep healthy and how to improve health; how to give advice on health matters to other people; how to avoid accidents, and how to cope in emergencies.

Element 1.1 looks at ways of improving health by health promotion, and examines the choices of lifestyle which will not put an individual at risk. The second element expands on this to ask you to produce a plan which will improve other people's health, and also to decide on the most effective way to give advice on health. The third element examines health hazards and how to avoid accidents. You will look at basic first aid skills which will enable you to cope with life-threatening health emergencies.

Element 1.1

Investigate Personal Health

unit one

Performance Criteria		
pc 1	Explain the importance of a balanced lifestyle	19
pc 2	Explain risks and benefits associated with aspects of lifestyle	20
pc 3	Identify how the body uses each dietary component	22
pc 4	Describe a healthy diet for an individual	24
pc 5	Describe the effects of use of substances on health and well-being	26
pc 6	Explain good practice in maintaining hygiene	28
	Summary of evidence opportunities and their relationship to the pcs	34
	Summary of element range and personal evidence tracking record	34

Introduction

This element is about general health matters.

You will learn the ways in which the health of individuals can be improved regardless of age, ability, or way of life. You will also learn how to encourage your clients to follow a healthy lifestyle so that their health can be maintained and they do not harm themselves by doing things which might damage their bodies or minds.

The element lays down the foundation knowledge for you to move on to Element 1.2, in which you will be learning how to pass on the information included here to other people.

Performance Criterion 1

The Importance of a Balanced Lifestyle

Our bodies and minds are designed to work as a whole; one affects the other.

We are constantly changing due to the influence of our own internal body systems, for example, our hormones, our response to illness, and ageing. We are also influenced by things outside ourselves, for example, the behaviour of other people, demands of work, and accidents. These changes mean that our bodies and minds have to be constantly adjusting in order to maintain a balance in our lives, whether the changes are enjoyable or unpleasant. Ideally, lifestyles are balanced in terms of

activity – work and recreation

rest – sleep and inactivity.

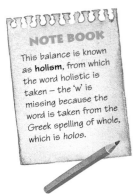

NOTE BOOK

This balance is known as **holism**, from which the word holistic is taken – the 'w' is missing because the word is taken from the Greek spelling of whole, which is holos.

ACTIVITY 1

1 Make a diagram illustrating the 'see-saw' of your own lifestyle, using the same factors as those in the diagram shown below. Do it in rough, so you can make the side go up and down if you think the importance of one activity is weightier than another. You will make a final copy later on.

2 Conduct a survey among colleagues to see what they regard as the most important factors contributing to positive health. Present the information in a graphical way. [NUM 2.1, 2.3]

The more we know about the needs for **positive health**, the easier it becomes to juggle with changes when the need arises.

Positive health

Positive health means more than good health, which could be taken to mean just the absence of ill health. Positive health is possible for everyone, whatever their age, even when they have a persistent or incurable illness, have problems understanding things, or have a physical disability. In your work you may have to give careful advice to your clients, as they could have difficulty understanding how to reach a balance in their lives. If all goes well, they will achieve a state of well-being. It is to do with accepting who we are, managing our lives effectively, and selecting a lifestyle which will help us to develop positive health.

Look at the see-saw diagram. Neither side is better than the other. It is all a matter of balancing the factors affecting lifestyle effectively for each individual.

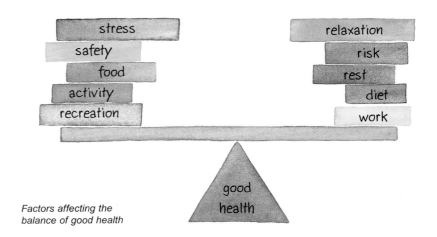

Factors affecting the balance of good health

Performance Criterion 2

Risks and Benefits Associated with Aspects of Lifestyles

Any lifestyle which excludes any of the needs listed below might place the individual's health at risk.

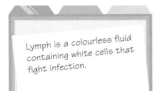

Lymph is a colourless fluid containing white cells that fight infection.

Needs for positive health

1 **Exercise**. The body benefits from exercise by

- improving muscle tone

- keeping the blood and lymphatic circulation moving

- increasing lung capacity

- keeping joints mobile

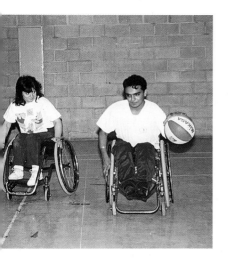

- helping digestion

- preventing constipation

- promoting well-being and reducing depression.

Exercise needs to be balanced with rest. An active child needs to have periods of quiet during which active muscles can recover. A person in a wheelchair needs to do regular exercises to counteract long hours sitting still.

Fitness and exercise are not concerned with the number of press-ups people can do or how far they can jog, but more with the strength and flexibility of their bodies. They are affected by an individual's

- state of health and presence of illness or disability

- age

- weight

- lung efficiency

- exercise levels and physical agility

- personality and attitude.

2 **A balanced diet** – contains the nutrients in the right proportions to maintain body health.
(Diet is discussed in detail in pc 3.)

3 **Sufficient rest** – allows the body and mind to recover after activity. In some cultures it is called 'allowing the soul to catch up'.

4 **Not smoking** – maintains the lungs in a clean condition and greatly reduces the possibility of bronchitis, lung cancer and heart disease in the smoker and other people.

5 **Avoidance of alcohol abuse** A sensible approach to drinking alcohol prevents dependency, liver and brain deterioration and the possibility of breakdown of relationships. It is generally thought that small amounts of alcohol are not harmful to the body.

6 **Safe sexual behaviour, including celibacy** A responsible attitude to sexual behaviour lessens the likelihood of contracting diseases such as Aids, hepatitis B, genital warts, herpes, gonorrhea, and cervical cancer.

Safe sexual behaviour includes:

- paying attention to personal hygiene after sex

- not having many sexual partners

- using a condom. This applies to heterosexual and homosexual partners

- celibacy, which means not having sexual relationships at all.

ACTIVITY 2

Return to the rough copy of your lifestyle which you made in Activity 1 and see if it needs adjusting. Make a good copy for your portfolio; it will provide evidence to demonstrate that you have thought about the importance of a balanced lifestyle.

Selecting an appropriate lifestyle

The lifestyle chosen by individuals tells us much about their personality and philosophy of living. However, not everyone can choose where they work or live, and this can cause stress and dissatisfaction when there is conflict between the dream of how they would like to live and the reality of their situation.

How balanced is your lifestyle?

Do you ever give yourself treats?

Is your working life satisfactory?

Does your work expand into your home life?*

Is your emotional life good?

How are your money matters?

Are you living where you want to?

Is your way of life healthy?

*Remember that 'work' includes study, and voluntary as well as paid work.

Are your treats good for you?

Do you get what you want from your holidays?

Do you enjoy your leisure time?

Could you spend more time with the people you care about?

Are you claiming all your benefits?

Could you improve your living space?

Would you feel happier if you ate/drank/exercised differently?

Performance Criterion 3

How the Body Uses each Dietary Component

Components

Food is principally made up of proteins, carbohydrates, fat, vitamins and minerals, water, and fibre. Most of us give little thought to these and concentrate on what we like or what is available. When you look after other people, however, you need to understand about the make up of food, as you may be called upon to provide low fat, low salt, high fibre, or other specialist diets.

Protein is what we are made of. It is the building material of our bodies. As our cells are constantly dying and being replaced – more quickly during some illnesses – protein is essential for us to flourish, grow and repair damaged tissues.

Carbohydrates provide the fuel for us to work. It was once thought that they alone caused people to put on weight. However, individuals who use a lot of energy need to eat carbohydrates to replace the energy that has been burnt up. Carbohydrates are divided into starches and sugars. All carbohydrates have to be converted into glucose before they can be used by the body. This process takes longer for starches than sugars. They take longer to digest and are more useful in stopping people from becoming hungry.

Fats are provided from animal or vegetable sources. The ones associated with harming the body by increasing the cholesterol level mostly come from animals, and are known as **saturated fats**. In general, vegetable fats are less harmful to our bodies when eaten in quantity, and are mostly known as **unsaturated fats**.

Fats provide twice the energy of carbohydrates and help proteins to carry out growth and repair, so while a low fat diet is a healthy one, the body could not function if fats were excluded altogether.

Vitamins and minerals Minute amounts of vitamins and minerals are needed to help the work of the proteins, carbohydrates and fats. Some minerals are important in themselves. Calcium builds up the structure of our bones and teeth. Iron maintains the health of our red blood cells. An ordinary balanced diet contains adequate vitamins and minerals. It is only when there are greater demands on the body, such as pregnancy or illness, that the average daily amounts need to be supplemented.

Fresh food is the best source of vitamins, as they deteriorate during storage or careless cooking. Vitamin C is found in fresh fruit and vegetables. It is important for the health of our skin, and helps the healing process in the body.

Vitamin D comes from fatty foods like margarine, eggs and fish containing fats. It is also made by our skin during exposure to sunlight. It is essential for healthy bones and teeth.

Water If we were squeezed dry, more than half of our bodies would be found to be made of water. Much of our body systems' energy is spent keeping the water and the nutrients dissolved in it in the right place. The balance is affected by our fluid intake and output, which changes with the body's temperature and that of the surroundings, and the amount of exercise taken. So we perspire and need to drink more when we are hot or exercising, and pass more urine when we are cold or resting.

The general requirement for fluid intake is about 1–1.5 litres (2 to 3 pints) daily. We **gain fluids** from all that we drink and much that we eat, and **lose fluids** by breathing, sweating and passing urine, and to a lesser extent, faeces.

Some substances increase the passing of urine. These are called **diuretics**. Caffeine is one, alcohol is another, and there are several medicines prescribed for people with fluid retention problems. Remember that fat cells contain very little water, so diuretics alone will not help in weight reduction. The table looks at factors affecting fluid loss.

Factors affecting fluid loss

+ = increased
– = decreased

	Body's response		
Factor	*urine output*	*sweating*	*thirst*
heat	-	+	+
cold	+	-	-
exercise	-	+	+
raised body temperature	-	+	+
diuretics	+	+	*normal*

Fibre

Fibre used to be called roughage, and was valued mainly in preventing constipation. Now it is also thought to give protection against diseases of the large intestine, and to help in lowering the amount of cholesterol in the blood.

Performance Criterion 4

A Healthy Diet for an Individual

Eating patterns

Our eating habits are affected by subtle psychological influences. We learn them from our families, friends, and the society in which we live. We use food as a bribe, as a reward, or as a treat or to comfort ourselves, as much as to satisfy hunger. Healthy eating has as much to do with our acceptance of ourselves as we are as it has to do with knowing the nutrients included in meals. Our appetites are often controlled by our emotions rather than our bodies' needs. Good carers never forget this when advising people about food, diet and feeding habits.

The table lists good and bad habits which contribute to a healthy diet.

Eating habits

GOOD HABITS	BAD HABITS
• keeping food out of sight between meals • not cooking too much, allowing for reasonable portions only • sitting down to eat • keeping to proper mealtimes • using minimal salt in cooking • keeping junk food out of the house	• smothering food with salt and relishes • finishing leftovers • using food for reward, or love substitute • eating on the move • 'grazing' continuously • bingeing then fasting • too much junk food

Healthy eating around the world

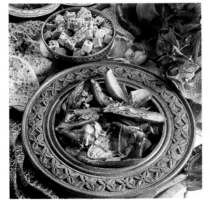

The Caribbean

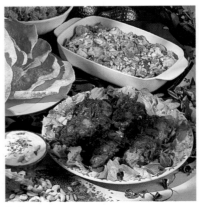

India

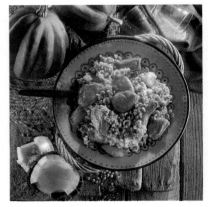

The Middle East

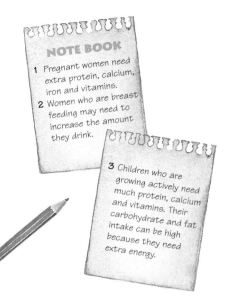

NOTE BOOK

1 Pregnant women need extra protein, calcium, iron and vitamins.

2 Women who are breast feeding may need to increase the amount they drink.

3 Children who are growing actively need much protein, calcium and vitamins. Their carbohydrate and fat intake can be high because they need extra energy.

Types of food eaten

- **proteins** such as meat, fish, dairy produce, pulses
- **carbohydrates** from starches such as potatoes, bread and pasta rather than sugars
- not too much **fat**, especially saturated animal fat
- **vitamins**, **minerals** and **fibre** from fresh fruit and vegetables
- **fibre** from whole foods, which tend to be 'brown' e.g. brown rice, brown wholemeal bread, brown flour
- not too much **salt** – do not add much during cooking, do not sprinkle it on after cooking
- not too much **sugar** or sweet food
- plenty of **fluids**, but not too much caffeine from tea or coffee (water is quite nice …)
- not too much **instant food and drink** – they contain additives and have lost much of their food value during preparation.

Amount eaten – See Activity 3.

Recommended daily intake of foods for an adult (see also Department of Health recommended diet - pie chart page 38)

Protein
half pint/250ml of milk
1 egg
average serving of: cheese, fish, nuts, peas, beans, lentils, meat

Carbohydrate
starches – freely but not in excess
sugars – only enough to make food enjoyable

Fruits and vegetables
3 to 5 servings

Water
at least 1 pint/500ml

Fats
only enough to make food enjoyable
 a animal fats • meat
              • butter and some hard margarines
              • full fat dairy produce

 b vegetable fats • sunflower oil
                • vegetable margarine

 c made-up foods • crisps
               • cakes
               • biscuits
               • chocolate

ACTIVITY 3

◀▶ Extension opportunity

1 Find out the daily intake of food recommended by the following bodies:
- NACNE – the National Advisory Committee on Nutrition Education
- COMA – the Committee on Medical Aspects of Food Policy
- JACNE – the Department of Health and the Joint Advisory Committee on Nutritional Education.

2 State how you found the information.

3 Record what you discover.
Diet breakdown can be illustrated effectively using percentages, fractions and decimal fractions. Use numerical information when you record this activity. [NUM 2.2]

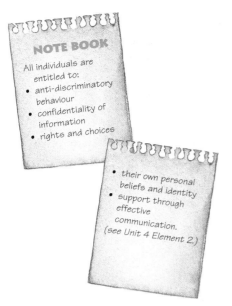

NOTE BOOK

All individuals are entitled to:
- anti-discriminatory behaviour
- confidentiality of information
- rights and choices

- their own personal beliefs and identity
- support through effective communication.
(See Unit 4 Element 2.)

Performance Criterion 5

What is an individual?

A dictionary definition of the word 'individual' is 'single, having distinct character'. When we talk about people as being individuals, we acknowledge that there is something special and distinctive about each one of them.

Individuals in society are of all ages – babies, children, adolescents, adults, those in mid-life, and older people. They will all have their own personalities – kind, grumpy, quiet, boisterous or dramatic, etc. They may be pregnant. They may be in good health or be ill, be very academic or rather practical, physically fit or physically disabled. Their way of life may be active or sedentary (which means sitting down), exciting or boring, rewarding or demanding.

All of them will be a mixture of age, personality, health status and way of life and will need to be respected accordingly by those whom they meet. You too are an individual and will have your own needs.

The Effects of Use of Substances on Health and Well-Being

Any substance taken into the body will have an effect on it. The effect may be

- physical
- social
- emotional
- intellectual.

Substances may be natural or manufactured. We will be examining drugs intended for use in medical treatment, misuse of drugs intended for use in medical treatment, use of drugs which have no intended use in medical treatment, and misuse of solvents.

ACTIVITY 4

Read through the following list of the possible effects of misusing substances:

- contracting diseases such as hepatitis B and Aids which can be spread during intravenous injection of substances
- the break up of relationships with friends and family
- difficulty in coping with a job
- dependency – which means unable to manage without something

- exposure to the danger of taking to crime to pay for the habit
- destruction of brain cells
- change in mental state
- inability to exercise control over one's actions
- mood swings.

Decide whether they can be classed as physical, social, emotional, or intellectual effects.

Record your decision, to use when you come to the case studies in this element.

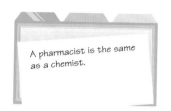

A pharmacist is the same as a chemist.

unit one

Drugs intended as medical treatment

Drug is another word for medicine. There are many thousands of drugs. Some commonly used ones are cough mixture, aspirin, and digoxin (a medicine given to regulate the heartbeat).

Many people are kept well by taking drugs regularly – think about those with diabetes or epilepsy. It is all to do with balance. The dose is regulated by the severity of the person's condition and his or her body weight, and is decided by a medical practitioner in many cases, or written on the container of drugs bought over the counter. Pharmacists will always respond to requests for clarification. Too low a dose of prescribed drugs can be as dangerous as too high a dose.

Drugs can be given by

- inhalation
- injection
- rubbing into the skin
- enema or suppository (inserted into the back passage)
- orally (which means by mouth).

Drugs should never be shared and unused medication should be returned to the pharmacist.

Misuse of drugs intended as medical treatment

Some people become dependent on drugs originally prescribed for a limited length of time. Examples include sedatives prescribed to help people to sleep, tranquillisers to reduce anxiety, and stimulants to promote alertness.

Use of drugs which have no accepted use in medical treatment

Drugs such as cannabis, heroin, cocaine and ecstasy are not considered acceptable in western society. Their prolonged use is considered to be a danger to health and creates a dependency which is destructive to the abuser.

Misuse of solvents

Solvents are designed to strip paints, light cigarettes, fuel cars and glue things together, not to be inhaled into people's lungs. Nevertheless, some people have a dependency on sniffing such substances, which causes confusion, loss of control, depression and ultimately death of brain cells.

Misuse of drugs and solvents is always damaging, and can be fatal.

Performance Criterion 6

Good Practice in Maintaining Hygiene

The two important aspects of hygiene to consider are **personal** and **public**.

Personal hygiene

Keeping clean requires some motivation and effort. People with low esteem, or a mental illness such as depression, find it hard to raise the energy to wash, bathe and clean their clothes. Those who feel constantly tired or ill may give their personal hygiene a low priority. Often the most humble carer looks after the cleanliness of clients. This is a very privileged position, as during baths, hair washing, or other intimate tasks clients will often talk freely and share their deepest thoughts, especially if the carer is scrupulous about attention to their privacy, dignity and self-respect.

The aim of hygiene routines is to encourage people to be as clean as is needed for good health and to be as able as possible to maintain this themselves. The diagram below looks at the objectives of personal hygiene and the potential barriers to achieving these.

People who are confused or psychologically damaged may cling to old routines. Older people may prefer the warm cosiness of a bath to the colder but quicker option of a shower. The use of deodorants may not be understood. Toe nails may have become out of reach due to an expanding waistline or increasing joint stiffness. Moving about may be painful. If so, washing and dressing could be put off until after breakfast when the morning pain-killer may have been given and the body has had the chance to loosen up.

It is rare that washing the intimate parts of the body cannot be performed by clients themselves. If you need to do this, be business-like and gentle, always paying attention to personal modesty – your own and the client's – and dignity. If you are performing a bed bath with a colleague *never* make remarks or gestures that could be misinterpreted, even if your patient is unconscious. You can never guess what is being understood even when a person appears not to be aware – the sense of hearing is the last to leave a person's conscious mind.

All over washing keeps the skin healthy and can be achieved by
- bathing
- showering
- strip washing (washing all over at a hand basin)
- bed bathing (washing all over while in bed)

Look for signs of dryness, rashes and other skin abnormalities while you help people to wash.

Care of the hair means
- attention from a hairdresser
- washing
- trimming
- shaving
- removing unwanted hair
- dealing with head lice.

Care of the mouth means
- dental inspection
- a healthy diet
- brushing the teeth
- denture care
- keeping the mouth of an ill person fresh and clean.

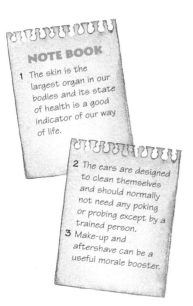

NOTE BOOK

1 The skin is the largest organ in our bodies and its state of health is a good indicator of our way of life.

2 The ears are designed to clean themselves and should normally not need any poking or probing except by a trained person.

3 Make-up and aftershave can be a useful morale booster.

personal preferences

incontinence

general hygiene needs

shyness

personal freshness

lack of mobility

healthy skin

cold bathrooms

bathing

damp towels

Objectives

Potential barriers

personal hygiene

Personal hygiene

Hygiene in public areas

Food hygiene

The **Food and Drugs Act 1955** and the **Food Hygiene (General) Regulations 1970** apply in all residential and nursing homes, and the manager is responsible for seeing that they are implemented. The basic rules will be displayed in the kitchen and should be followed by all staff.

The kitchen, both at home and at work, should be kept clean with hot soapy water, and tidied to reduce the risk of accidents. The table on the left gives a check list.

Eating areas

Dining areas, or personal trays, should be clean and attractive. Tray and table cloths will need washing often, as will table napkins if fabric ones are used. Cutlery should be shiny and crockery unchipped.

The floor will need sweeping or hoovering after each meal. Keep an eye open for tablets as these are often given out at mealtimes and may be unintentionally or intentionally dropped on to the floor.

Medical treatment areas

Medical treatment areas should be kept scrupulously clean. **Asepsis** means the absence of germs which can cause infection. It is impossible to achieve under normal conditions and therefore sterile disposable dressings are used to cover wounds whenever aseptic conditions are required. In addition to a clean environment:

- all surfaces should be clean and dry and all staff should wash and dry their hands thoroughly, both before and after treatment

- after use, all disposable equipment should be wrapped up, put into a bag and burnt

- sharp equipment should be put into a special yellow box labelled **'sharps'** and disposed of separately.

Kitchen hygiene

- perishable food should be kept in a refrigerator
- clean the refrigerator regularly
- protect food from flies
- dispose of food scraps quickly
- use bins with lids and empty them frequently
- dishcloths and mops should be rinsed out after use and left to dry
- wash dishes up in hot soapy water, rinse in hot water and leave to drain, then put them away in a cupboard or shelf
- wash up straight away or put dirty articles in the dishwasher rather than allow dirty dishes to pile up

unit one

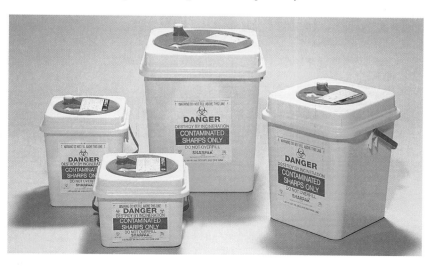

29

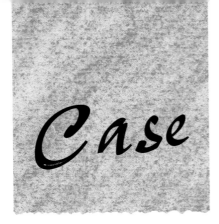

Case Studies

Before you start, make a reference list of

a the most important reasons for following a balanced way of life

b methods of reducing health risks

c the effects of substance and drug abuse on health and well-being (from Activity 4).

Then, using the information you have gathered together, respond to the case studies presented here.

Case study 2   Down Way School

Kevin is five, and has asthma. An inhaler is kept in the staff room for him to use before he plays football, which he loves, and which he plays very well. When Jalwinder hangs up his coat one day it smells strongly of stale cigarette smoke. Three empty crisp packets fall out of the pockets, which could explain why Kevin eats so little at lunch time.

Task 2

Write a report in which you consider the following issues:

1 If she had to discuss his health with his parents, how would Jalwinder explain

a why the school thinks it is important for him to continue to play football

Case study 1   The Thatched Cottage

Eileen is a recent arrival. Before admission, she had lived alone in a cold flat, not eating properly, and having no inclination to wash or change her clothes. She enjoys it in The Thatched Cottage, being warm and having her food prepared for her. She snoozes comfortably in an armchair most of the day.

She is now finding it difficult to sleep through the night and is beginning to put on weight. She admits that she is becoming lazy about hygiene, but 'can't see the point' now that she is no longer responsible for her own washing and cleaning. She has agreed with Mark to help him with his college coursework.

Task 1

1 How could Mark work out what could have happened to the balance of Eileen's lifestyle which would cause these changes?

2 How might he demonstrate this with a before and after see-saw?

Task 1

3 How could he explain to Eileen why a balanced lifestyle is important?

Mention of fractions could be appropriate here. Display any numerical calculations which you have made. [NUM 2.1, 2.2]

Task 1

4 What are the most important aspects of good practice in personal hygiene which might help to motivate Eileen?

5 Using images – either drawn or with a computer – explain the importance of hygienic practices in one of the public areas of The Thatched Cottage.

Task 2

b the effect of cigarette smoke on his state of health

c other ways of reducing health risks in general

Use of graphical information could highlight problems associated with smoking. [NUM 2.3]

Case study 3 Netherfield Community Care

Debbie's aunt works in the local doctor's surgery, and knows that she is following a course in Health and Social Care. She becomes friendly with Jane, a patient who has ME (Mylagic encephalomyelitis, which causes severe fatigue over a long period of time), and is pregnant. She wants to help Jane to eat well during her pregnancy, and is also concerned that James, her young son, should eat sensibly. Jane's grandmother lives next door, and often gives James sweets and chocolates.

Debbie's aunt suggests that Debbie should make out a list for Jane of the foods which would be of benefit to her, James and her grandmother. The list is to help with the shopping, and also with a typical day's menu for all three individuals. Jane is interested to know why each of the foods recommended is good for their health, and how much of it they should eat.

Task 3

1 Produce the sort of list that Debbie might make for a day's menu for all three individuals. Write beside each food how it is used by the body and indicate the amount of that food component that should be eaten each day.

Task 3

Mention of percentages, ratios and average indicators would help to emphasise the benefits of a healthy diet. Amounts could be expressed in decimal fractions.

[num 2.1, 2.2]

Case study 4 Hill Hall

Many of the children are dependent on medication to make their lives tolerable. Danny is a new boy. His mother has become interested in herbal remedies and wants to discuss discontinuing his prescribed drugs and substituting others which her daughter finds helpful. The staff are talking about this over coffee. Some sympathise with the mother's view, others disagree with her.

Task 4

Discuss in a group

a how prescribed drugs might be helping Danny

b possible results of discontinuing them

c with whom it would be appropriate for Danny's mother to discuss the changes she desires

Task 4

d possible consequences of sharing another person's medication, either conventional or herbal.

unit one case studies

31

Multiple Choice Questions

1 Which person has the greatest need of protein in the diet?

    a *an eight-year-old child*

    b *a middle-aged man*

    c *an elderly woman*

    d *a thirty-year-old woman*

2 Which of the following is *most* likely to be affected by inadequate body hygiene?

    a *dietary intake*

    b *intellectual development*

    c *personal activities*

    d *physical health*

3 When a person spends a long time sitting down, his or her lifestyle is described as being

    a *passive*

    b *mobile*

    c *sedentary*

    d *active*

4 Decide which of these statements about food is true (T) and which is false (F).

    a *plenty of salt is good for you*

    b *fibre makes you fat*

    c *food can be a substitute for love*

    d *you feel less hungry for longer after eating potatoes than after eating sweets*

    e *people should drink less as they grow older*

5 Drug abuse means that

    a *vitamin supplements are taken unnecessarily*

    b *tranquillisers are taken regularly*

    c *prescribed drugs are taken in recommended doses*

    d *drugs are taken which have no accepted use in medical treatment*

6 Which of the following is a health risk?

    a *a vegetarian eating beans instead of meat*

    b *a housewife drinking a glass of red wine each evening*

    c *a person with diabetes taking less insulin than the prescribed dose*

    d *a child climbing a tree*

7 Fats in the diet are used by the body to

    a *repair tissues*

    b *provide energy*

    c *convert glucose*

    d *prevent constipation*

8 Which *one* of the following phrases *best* describes a balanced diet?

    a *food is eaten only when a person is hungry*

    b *adequate protein is taken to repair damaged cells*

    c *all food components are taken in adequate quantities*

    d *food intake is sufficient to maintain body weight*

CROSSWORD 'Food for thought'

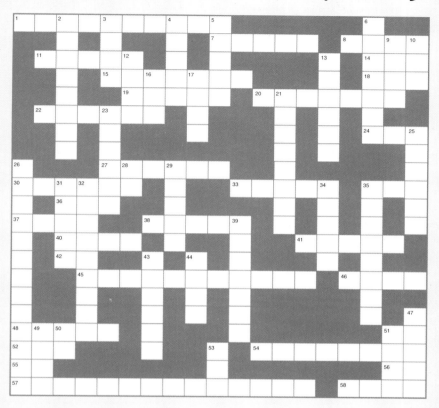

Across

1 Naughty but nice   5, 5
7 What you pay for food   5
8 Not recommended in excess   4
11 Sooner or later it may settle on the bottom!   5
14 A star sign   3
15 Contains nicotine   7
18 It contains preserved food   3
19 Families eat their meals from it   5
20 The body builder   7
22 Description of someone whose religion prohibits the eating of pork   6
24 Does it gather germs in the sink?   3
27 We shouldn't do this between meals   6
30 Do they keep the doctor away?   6
33 A mother does this when she gets her baby used to solid food   5
35 None on food   3
36 Meat less good for you than white   3
37 Comes from cows   4
38 Angry action for teeth?   5
40 A way to fry   4
41 Someone who eats no animal products   5
42 Thus   2

45 People who eat no meat   11
46 Can be made from sunflowers, nuts and olives   4
48 Not quite right   5
51 Fourth note of scale   2
52 Green bottles?   3
54 6 down is one of the essential ones   8
55 A prefix   2
56 Describes position   2
57 Types of 26 down   5, 3, 6
58 We cook in them   4

Down

2 Code letters for additives   1, 7
3 Source of animal protein   4
4 Turkish way of serving food   5
5 Variety is the – – – – – of life   5
6 Essential for strong teeth and bones   7
9 Contains little fat   3
10 A measure of weight seldom used in cooking!   3
12 Food does this if not kept cool in hot weather   4
13 Lancashire stew   6
16 Expression of disgust   3

17 Can result from hardening of the arteries   4
21 Is now known as fibre   8
23 Pressed   6
25 Causes jam to set   6
26 Give us energy   13
28 State of being   2
29 Runners, jumping or black eyed!   5
31 Squeeze   5
32 Eating too many puts on weight   4-5
34 Does the thought of mint sauce frighten them?   5
35 Supplements not always necessary   8
39 State of cleanliness desirable in the kitchen   7
43 Source of vegetable protein   6
44 Food provided   4
47 Doesn't eat   5
49 Bill of fare   4
50 Contained   2
51 An open tart   4
53 Essential for health – but don't eat too much   3

Summary of Evidence Opportunities and their Relationship to Performance Criteria

Activities 1 and 2 pcs 1 and 2	**Case study 1** pcs 1, 2 and 6	**Case study 4** pc 5
Activity 3 pc 4	**Case study 2** pc 2	
Activity 4 pc 5	**Case study 3** pcs 3 and 4	

Unit 1 Element 1 Summary of Element Range and Personal Evidence Tracking Record

Element range references (tick against left-hand column)	Description of evidence	Pc and range covered	Portfolio reference number
Pc 1 Lifestyle balance			
activity – work			
– recreation			
rest – sleep			
– inactivity			
Pc 2 Aspects of lifestyle			
exercise			
diet – adequate			
– balanced			
sufficient rest			
smoking			
alcohol			
sexual behaviour including celibacy			
Pc 3 Dietary components			
components – protein			
– carbohydrate			
– fat			
– vitamins C and D			
– minerals, iron and calcium			
– water			
– fibre			
Pc 4 Healthy diet			
types of food eaten			
amount eaten			
eating patterns			
Individuals			
active			
sedentary			
child			
elderly person			
pregnant woman			

Unit 1 Element 1 Summary of Element Range and Personal Evidence Tracking Record			
Element range references *(tick against left-hand column)*	**Description of evidence**	**Pc and range covered**	**Portfolio reference number**
Pc 5 Substances			
use of drugs intended as medical treatment			
misuse of drugs intended as medical treatment			
use of drugs with no accepted use in medical treatment			
misuse of solvents			
Effects of substances			
physical			
social			
emotional			
intellectual			
Pc 6 Hygiene			
personal – teeth			
– skin			
– hair			
public areas – food preparation			
– eating			
– medical treatment			

unit one

Element 1.2

Present Advice on Health and Well-Being to Others

Performance Criteria

pc 1 Assess an individual's health against standard measures   36

pc 2 Produce a plan to improve an individual's health   41

pc 3 Produce advice on maintaining health and well-being, related to the needs of a target group   43

pc 4 Present the advice to the target group   43

pc 5 Assess the impact of the advice on the target group   45

Summary of evidence opportunities and their relationship to the pcs   49

Summary of element range and personal evidence tracking record   49

Introduction

This element is about advising other people how to adapt their habits in order to improve their way of life. You will learn about the general recommendations currently laid down for good health, so that you have definite standards against which you can measure someone's present lifestyle. This of course, includes your own.

Performance Criterion 1

Assess an Individual's Health Against Standard Measures

You can assess someone's health in terms of exercise, diet, sleep and rest and other factors related to the individual, using standard measures of food tables, fitness measures, and physical measures.

Exercise

When working out how much exercise a person takes each day, we need to take into consideration the ordinary activities of his or her daily life: for instance, walking upstairs, walking to the shops or work, cycling, housework, looking after a toddler, gardening, or operating a wheelchair or frame. All of these help to keep the heart and lungs healthy, which is called **cardiovascular fitness**. An increase in everyday activities is to be encouraged before someone is recommended to take up a sport. It can be harmful for an unfit person to undertake sudden strenuous activity.

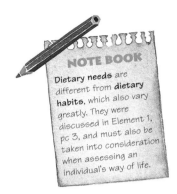

NOTE BOOK

Dietary needs are different from dietary habits, which also vary greatly. They were discussed in Element 1, pc 3, and must also be taken into consideration when assessing an individual's way of life.

The benefits of being fit are felt after any increase in exercise, such as walking, cycling, jogging, dancing, swimming, badminton, or football. All of these are examples of **aerobic exercise**, which is the most beneficial for cardiovascular fitness.

Diet

People's dietary needs vary greatly according to

- age – young children need more protein than adults
- mode of life – active or sedentary
- state of health
- personal metabolism – the rate at which energy is burned up
- personal dietary needs – they may need a special diet to keep them in good health, for example, people with diabetes.

Sleep and rest

Individual needs for sleep vary; babies sleep a great deal, gradually requiring less sleep as they grow older. Older people generally sleep less than young adults.

Relaxation

As we grow older we tend to sleep less, but our need for relaxation and rest increases. Young children need opportunities to recover from running about and other physical activities necessary to the healthy development of their bodies. Everybody needs relaxation for the mind and brain to recover from mental and emotional activities.

New born baby	20
Infant	12
Child	10
Adult	8
Older person	7

At all ages individual needs vary according to temperament and level of physical activity.

Average hours of sleep needed

Factors related to the individual

All the following will affect people's inclination or ability to act on advice about their general level of health:

- general health and level of fitness
- presence of illness
  - short term (e.g. measles)
  - long term (e.g. asthma)
- mental health (for example, the client may be schizophrenic)
- level of understanding (for example, the client may be autistic)
- gender and age – women tend to respond to health advice more readily than men. Younger men tend to respond to health advice more readily than older men.

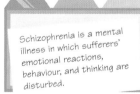

Schizophrenia is a mental illness in which sufferers' emotional reactions, behaviour, and thinking are disturbed.

Autism is a condition in which the sufferer is unable to relate to people, and is often disturbed by change.

Standard measures of health

Food tables

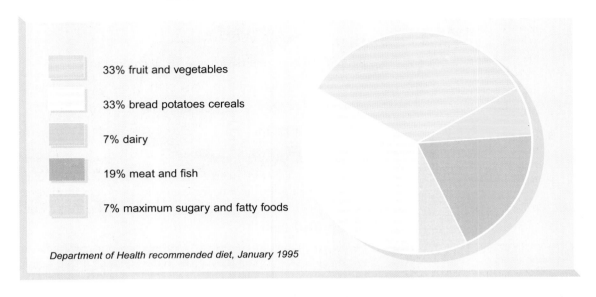

33% fruit and vegetables

33% bread potatoes cereals

7% dairy

19% meat and fish

7% maximum sugary and fatty foods

Department of Health recommended diet, January 1995

Fitness measures

Taking the pulse rate into account is an easy and effective way of measuring people's fitness levels. It is a good indicator of heart and circulation fitness. Activity 1 and the table below look at measuring **pulse rates** and Activity 2 looks at measuring **lung efficiency**.

Age group	Resting			After activity *		
	Young	Middle	Elderly	Young	Middle	Elderly
Men						
Good	60 – 70	65 – 72	68 – 75	76 – 84	80 – 88	84 – 90
Average	70 – 85	72 – 87	76 – 90	85 – 100	88 – 104	92 – 104
Poor	86+	88+	90+	102+	104+	106+
Women						
Good	72 – 77	72 – 79	77 – 83	88 – 92	88 – 94	92 – 98
Average	78 – 95	80 – 98	84 – 102	99 – 110	95 – 114	100 – 116
Poor	96+	99+	103+	112+	114+	118+

* For example, running on the spot for 1 minute.

Safe maximum pulse rate			
Age group	Young	Middle	Elderly
	170	155	140

The pulse should not exceed these rates during exercise.

Analysis of average pulse rates

ACTIVITY 1

1 Take your own pulse when you have not been active for sometime. Repeat, this time with the pulse of a friend. Take the measure at the wrist or the neck.

2 Repeat after exercise (e.g. running on the spot for one minute; climbing stairs)

3 Compile the information in a table, then present it using a variety of graphical methods.

[NUM 2.1, 2.3, 2.2]

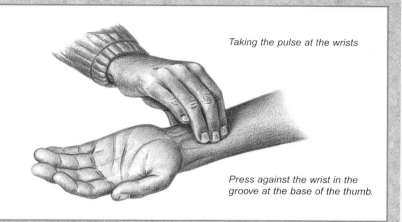

Taking the pulse at the wrists

Press against the wrist in the groove at the base of the thumb.

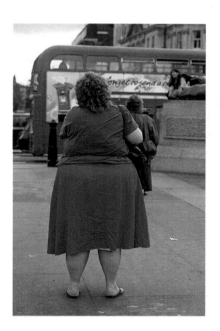

Physical measures

Weight and **body fat** are useful physical measures. A health survey for England published in 1993 showed evidence that adults were getting fatter despite national health education campaigns.

Body mass index   The standard measure of weight is the **body mass index**, or BMI. To work out your body mass index you take the weight in kilograms and divide it by the square of your height in metres.

$$\textbf{BMI} = \frac{\text{weight (kg)}}{\text{height (m)} \times \text{height (m)}}$$

A BMI of 30 or more means you are dangerously overweight, or **obese**.

A BMI of 25–30 means you are overweight.

The table on p.40 shows recommended height/weight ratios as advised by the Health Education Authority.

ACTIVITY 2

How efficient are your lungs?

1 Time how long you can hold your breath – it should be 45 seconds or more.

2 Measure your chest when you have breathed in and again after breathing out. The difference should be 5–7 cms.

3 What would this be in inches? [NUM 2.2 pc7]

These measures can be used with clients to see if breathing exercises would improve their lung capacity.

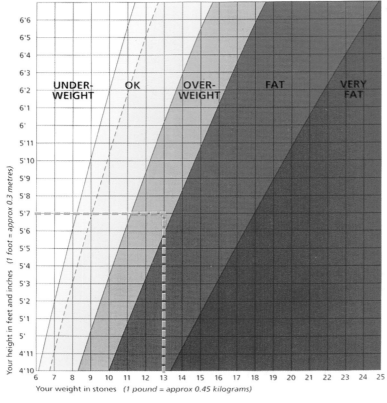

Recommended height/weight ratios (Health Education Authority)

Chart labels: UNDER-WEIGHT, OK, OVER-WEIGHT, FAT, VERY FAT

Y-axis: Your height in feet and inches *(1 foot = approx 0.3 metres)*

X-axis: Your weight in stones *(1 pound = approx 0.45 kilograms)*

ACTIVITY 3

1 Measure the height and weight of a range of people.

2 Present the information using a variety of graphical methods.

3 Summarise the information displayed by using appropriate representative values – e.g. median.

4 Measure the BMI of each individual showing your calculations. **[NUM 2.1, 2.3, 2.2]**

5 Enter this information into a spreadsheet and select an appropriate graphing method to display it – e.g. pie chart, bar chart. **[IT 2.1, 2.2, 2.3]**

ACTIVITY 4

Working in pairs:

1 Breath out and relax.

2 Measure waist.

3 Breath in.

4 Measure chest when lungs are full.

5 Work out the difference between the two measurements, displaying all numerical calculations when reaching conclusions drawn from results.

6 If you have worked in imperial measures (inches), convert your result into metric measures (centimetres) – and vice versa. **[NUM 2.2]**

If the waist measurement is greater than the chest measurement, there is a need to lose weight.

Extension opportunity

1 Think about a person you know well, who feels that their personal health or well-being would benefit from attention.

2 Find some standard measure(s) of health and well-being other than those explained above, which would be relevant to this person.

3 Assess the individual's health against the measure(s).

4 Make a record of the procedure you have undertaken. Remember the confidentiality issues.

If you are able to gain the person's consent and approval, you could make this a real exercise. Otherwise it will have to be theoretical.

Performance Criterion 2

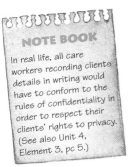

NOTE BOOK

In real life, all care workers recording clients' details in writing would have to conform to the rules of confidentiality in order to respect their clients' rights to privacy. (See also Unit 4, Element 3, pc 5.)

Produce a Plan to Improve an Individual's Health

In Unit 1, Element 1 you learnt about the needs for positive health. In the first part of this element you learnt some of the ways of measuring an individual's state of health. Now you will learn how to draw up a plan to help someone to lead a more healthy life, beginning with an assessment, from which an action plan will be devised.

The action plan

An action plan has to consider the priorities for action, that is, their order of importance. The personal targets that the client hopes to achieve in the short and long term need to be thought through and followed by a reassessment of the targets. Do the targets need to be changed?

unit one

Plan for living

1 Assessment

Name ....   Date ....

a Present state of health	Good	Acceptable	Poor		Good	Acceptable	Poor
Physical fitness				Taking of prescribed			
Diet				medication (if applicable)			
Hygiene				Rest/relaxation			
Smoking				Substance abuse			
Alcohol consumption				Drug dependency			

Anything appearing in the *'poor'* column needs carrying on to the next chart.
You will guess that some of the topics will need tactful discussion.

b Risks to health

Level of risk	No risk	Low - not dangerous			High - dangerous	
	0	1	2	3	4	5
Level of physical exercise						
Diet						
Hygiene						
Smoking						
Alcohol consumption						
Taking of prescribed medication (if applicable)						
Rest/relaxation						
Substance abuse						
Drug dependency						

c Factors to be considered (circle as applicable)

General health   *Good*   *Average*   *Poor*   *if poor, explain*

Presence of illness   short term   state cause ....

                      long term   state cause ....

Mental health   *Good*   *Average*   *Poor if poor, explain*

Level of understanding *explain*

2 Action plan

Things which need to be improved	Ways of improving them	Order of importance

Targets	What the client hopes to achieve:	What the benefits will be:
a short term		
b long term		

Appraisal
Have the things in the first list improved?
Do the targets need to be changed?
If so, in what way?

Date

ACTIVITY 5

Continue with Case study 2 from Element 1.1 (see page 30).

1 Using the table above as a model, draw up an assessment plan for Kevin, adapting the model where you feel it is necessary.

2 Devise an action plan from your findings.

ACTIVITY 6

1 Working in pairs, draw up an assessment plan for each of you to estimate where you need to improve your personal health.

2 When deciding on your targets, write down when these will be reviewed. Don't attempt too many changes. Your plan needs to be realistic

Performance Criterion 3

Produce Advice on Maintaining Health and Well-Being Related to the Needs of a Target Group

Carers often have to give health advice to groups of those they look after. These are called **target groups** and could be any of the following:

- children
- pregnant women
- elderly people
- those who are physically active
- those who are sedentary
- people with physical disabilities.

Sometimes individuals fit into more than one group.

ACTIVITY 7

1 Into which target groups would the clients in case studies 1–4 in Element 1.1 fit? (See pages 30–31.)

2 Record your findings

Performance Criterion 4

Present the Advice to the Target Group

We need to know which target group individuals fit into so that any health advice given can be set out in a way which is suitable for them, otherwise it will not be understood or acted upon. This is called its **presentation format**.

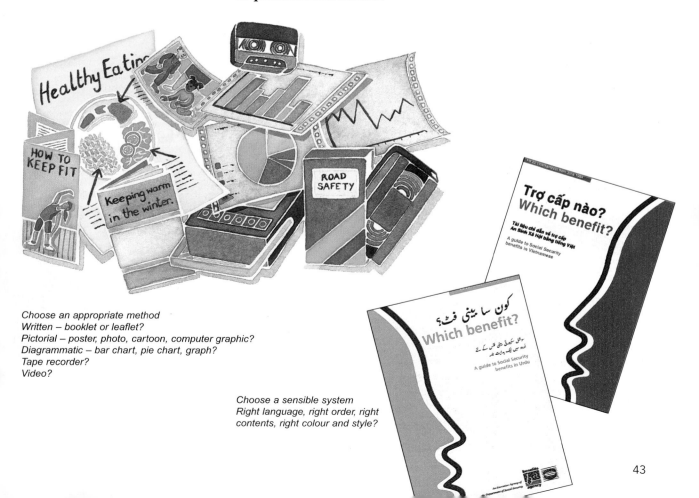

Choose an appropriate method
Written – booklet or leaflet?
Pictorial – poster, photo, cartoon, computer graphic?
Diagrammatic – bar chart, pie chart, graph?
Tape recorder?
Video?

Choose a sensible system
Right language, right order, right contents, right colour and style?

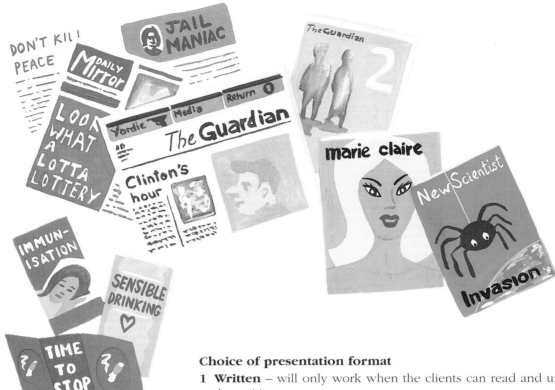

*Make sure of your information
Is it up-to-date? reliable? accurate?
Did I get it from a source I can trust?
Do I need to check it?*

Choice of presentation format

1 Written – will only work when the clients can read and understand the writing.

2 Diagrammatic – sometimes conveys the meaning more clearly than words.

3 Pictorial – it has been said that a picture saves a thousand words: sometimes a picture is more attractive than writing, often it is easier to understand.

4 Audio-visual – a good way to transmit complicated information and often suitable for groups.

The table below illustrates some of the factors which influence choice of format for presenting information to the target group.

Factors influencing choice of presentation format

DESIGN ASPECTS	PRACTICAL POINTS
• size and type of paper	• cost
• use of colour	• availability of material
• medium – paint, crayon, felt pen, etc.	• skills of team (if applicable)
• amount of space on the page	• own abilities
• colour of background	• distribution of finished presentation
• best layout – poster, booklet, leaflet, etc.	• time constraints

Performance Criterion 5

Assess the Impact of the Advice on the Target Group

After any work with clients, it is wise to spend time looking back to see how useful the activity has been. This is called **evaluation**. In this case you want to discover how effective your presentation has been, and whether or not your clients have acted on the advice you gave. Sometimes the effort seems to have no effect, and often the effect is difficult to measure, especially if the target group finds it hard to put thoughts into words because they are too young, too old, or too disabled to describe things using words.

Evaluation is carried out by getting **feedback** from the clients. You need to find out if the presentation format was appropriate, and if they intend to take notice of the information it contained.

This can be done by formal or informal methods.

Formal methods

Formal methods can take the form of a series of questions with responses. The responses could be **verbal**, or in a group discussion for formal review, or **written**, a simple tick or cross, 'smiley' faces showing degrees of pleasure and displeasure, or graded numbers.

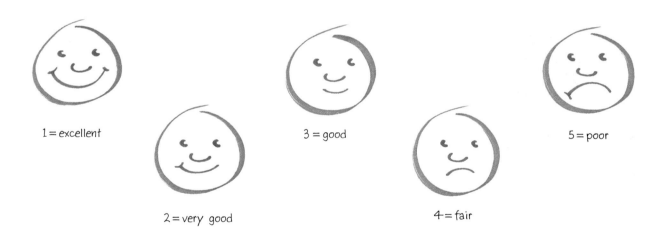

1 = excellent

2 = very good

3 = good

4 = fair

5 = poor

Informal methods

More informal methods of evaluation include:

- watching behaviour
- asking questions
- seeing if habits change
- listening for comments
- informal discussion.

The skill lies in selecting a method which can be easily used and understood by the client group involved. You will also have to decide whether your findings need to be recorded and/or reported to others.

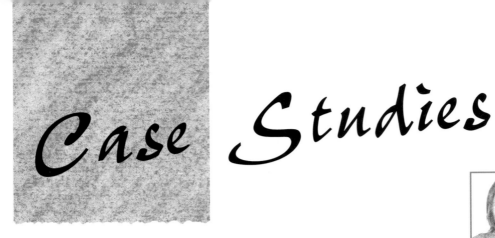

Case Studies

Case study 1   Hill Hall

There are four people with moderate learning difficulties living semi-independently in an annexe to Hill Hall school. It is suspected that someone has been climbing in over the wall and inhaling solvents in the back garden during the night. The residents are impressionable, so there is a danger that they could find and experiment with the debris that is left, or try to copy the habit. Molly discovers that Ann enjoys planning projects, and realises that this is an opportunity to help her to communicate with the clients in a very useful way.

Task 1

1   Molly asks Ann to design a health promotion package explaining to the residents of the hostel the dangers of substance abuse. Use the information in the text to help you decide on an appropriate presentation format.

Task 1

Then design the package that Ann might produce. The format should NOT be in poster form – you will be using this in Case study 3. You may decide to use a computer for this activity.
[COMM 2.2, 2.3; IT 2.1, 2.2, 2.3]

Task 1

2   How might Ann devise an appropriate method of evaluating the effectiveness of her advice?

Case study 2   The Thatched Cottage

Dora is going to aerobics classes and is feeling very fit and well. She wants to share her enthusiasm with the residents by encouraging them to take more exercise within their capabilities. She enlists Mark's help with some suitable music on his tape recorder, and the residents begin gentle exercises in their chairs.

Task 2

1   How could Dora and Mark work out the effectiveness of their scheme?
2   How long should they wait before assessing its value, and why?

Case study 3   Netherfield Community Care

Several young men live together in a hostel for people with physical disabilities. Different aids to mobility allow them to keep active, their kitchen is adapted for cooking, and they shop for one another in a nearby shopping precinct. They have asked Debbie and Mikhail to produce a poster to explain to them realistic ways of reducing health risks in their daily lives. They want it to look good as it is intended for their sitting room.

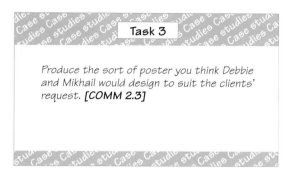

Task 3

Produce the sort of poster you think Debbie and Mikhail would design to suit the clients' request. **[COMM 2.3]**

Case study 4   Down Way School

Some of the children have been eating reluctantly at lunchtime. It is found that they have seen a television programme about reducing diets, and they have decided to slim. Isabel and Jalwinder want to do some work with the children about healthy eating and appropriate weight/height ratios for their age. The aim is to strengthen the work the teaching staff are doing with the parents about the children's lunches.

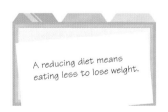

A reducing diet means eating less to lose weight.

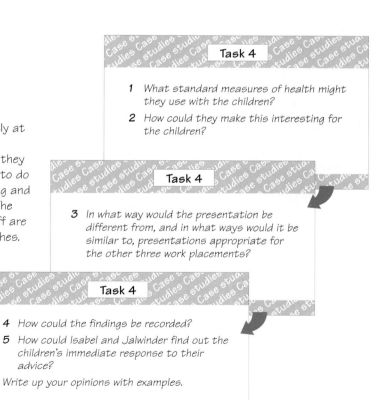

Task 4

1 What standard measures of health might they use with the children?

2 How could they make this interesting for the children?

Task 4

3 In what way would the presentation be different from, and in what ways would it be similar to, presentations appropriate for the other three work placements?

Task 4

4 How could the findings be recorded?

5 How could Isabel and Jalwinder find out the children's immediate response to their advice?

Write up your opinions with examples.

Multiple Choice Questions

1 Working out the state of a person's health is called

    a *acceptability*

    b *accreditation*

    c *assessment*

    d *evaluation*

2 Which of the following is a standard measure of health?

    a *protein/carbohydrate ratio*

    b *weight/height ratio*

    c *health/fitness ratio*

    d *sleep/relaxation ratio*

3 After carrying out a health promotion exercise, which of the following would show that your advice had been ignored?

    a *the client's habits would remain unchanged*

    b *the client's health would improve*

    c *the carers would feel less stressed*

    d *the carers' relations with the client would improve*

4 When things are prioritised, they are

    a *left unfinished*

    b *put in alphabetical order*

    c *put in order of importance*

    d *done immediately*

5 Which would be the *MOST* suitable method of promoting care of the teeth to a class of five year old children?

    a *a typed page of information*

    b *a formal lecture*

    c *a written quiz*

    d *a cartoon poster*

6 When assessing an elderly man's lifestyle, it is discovered that he enjoys late night television programmes. Which of the following effects would be considered a health risk?

    a *it causes him to go to bed late*

    b *it stops him from sleeping well*

    c *his wife disapproves*

    d *he seldom watches day-time television*

7 Which of the pie charts on p.49 illustrates best the recommended dietary components?

◀▶ **Extension opportunity**

You could record and present the pie charts in approximate percentages, fractions or decimal fractions. **[NUM]**

8 Which *one* of the following could be described as a long-term personal target for inclusion in a health plan?

    a *maintaining an exercise programme*

    b *assessing the individual's lifestyle*

    c *evaluating the effects of the plan*

    d *identifying priorities for action*

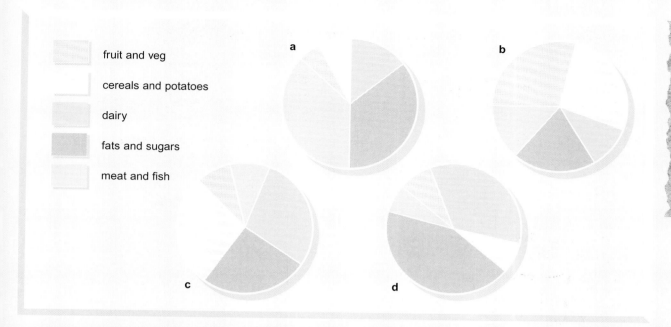

fruit and veg

cereals and potatoes

dairy

fats and sugars

meat and fish

a

b

c

d

Summary of Evidence Opportunities and their Relationship to Performance Criteria

Activities 1, 2, 3 and 4	pc 1	**Case study 1**	pcs 3 and 5	**Case study 4**	pcs 1, 3, 4 and 5
Activities 5 and 6	pc 2	**Case study 2**	pc 5		
Activity 7	pc 3	**Case study 3**	pc 4		

Unit 1 Element 1.2 Summary of Element Range and Personal Evidence Tracking Record

Element range references (tick against left-hand column)	Description of evidence	Pc and range covered	Portfolio reference number
Pc 1 Health assessed in terms of			
exercise			
diet			
sleep and rest			
other factors related to the individual			
Standard measures			
food tables			
fitness measures			
physical measures			
Pc 2 Health plan			
priorities for action			
personal targets – short term			
– long term			
reassessment of targets			

Unit 1 Element 1.2 Summary of Element Range and Personal Evidence Tracking Record

Element range references (*tick against left-hand column*)	Description of evidence	Pc and range covered	Portfolio reference number
Pc 3 Target group			
active			
sedentary			
children			
pregnant women			
elderly people			
people with disabilities			
Pc 4 Presentation formats			
written			
diagrammatic			
pictorial			
audio-visual			
Pc 5 Impact			
feedback on presentation			
response to advice			

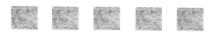

Element 1.3

Reduce Risk of Injury and Deal with Emergencies

Performance Criteria

pc 1   Explain hazards which could affect the health of individuals   51

pc 2   Describe methods of reducing risk of injury from hazards   51

pc 3   Describe personal roles and responsibilities in dealing with health emergencies   57

pc 4   Explain the physiological basis of basic life-saving techniques for dealing with health emergencies   59

pc 5   Demonstrate basic life-saving techniques in simulated health emergencies   62

Summary of evidence opportunities and their relationship to the pcs   71

Summary of element range and personal evidence tracking record   71

Introduction

The last element in this unit is designed to make you aware of hazards to health in the immediate surroundings (both indoors and outside) to help you to learn how to reduce the likelihood of accidents. It will also tell you how to deal with emergency situations by using basic life-saving skills.

Performance Criterion 1

Hazards which could Affect the Health of Individuals

Performance Criterion 2

Methods of Reducing Risk of Injury from Hazards

These two performance criteria are covered in the text together.

We are constantly surrounded by danger. Safety is to do with recognising dangers, or **hazards**, and keeping the risks they pose under control. Those who need looking after may not be able to recognise these hazards. So we must be on the alert to make sure that their surroundings are made as safe as possible without placing too many restrictions on individuals' independence.

The secret of reducing the risk of accidents is to use everything for its intended purpose, and to keep surroundings tidy. Muddle creates muddle and encourages muddled thinking. Fewer accidents happen in a tidy and controlled environment.

It is a sad fact that most accidents occur in people's own homes, so we need to begin by looking at safety right under our noses – in the home and garden, on the road, in social settings, and in the local environment.

Hazards in the home and garden

ACTIVITY 1

Look at the table and then draw connecting lines linking the hazard with the risk. One is done for you as an example.

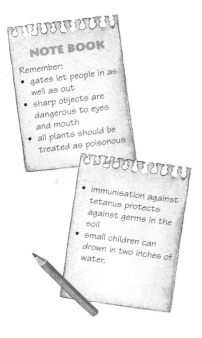

NOTE BOOK

Remember:
- gates let people in as well as out
- sharp objects are dangerous to eyes and mouth
- all plants should be treated as poisonous

- immunisation against tetanus protects against germs in the soil
- small children can drown in two inches of water.

a KITCHEN

RISK	HAZARD
Fire	Refrigerator
Burns and scalds	Hot pans
Cuts	Waste bin
Infection	Cleaning materials
Poisoning	Electrical equipment
Tripping/falling	Knives
Electrocution	Cooker
	Mats
	Spilt food

b BATHROOM

RISK	HAZARD
Scalding	Electrical equipment
Poisoning	Bath
Falling	Shampoo
Cuts	Water
Drowning	Lavatory
Infection	Tablets
Allergies	Flannels
Electrocution	Bath mats
	Soap/bubble bath
	Taps

c OTHER ROOMS

RISK	HAZARD
Falling	Ashtrays
Poisoning	Bottles of alcohol
Burns	Electrical equipment
Cuts	Poor lighting
Electrocution	Loose carpets
Fire	Toys left on the floor
Infection	Pets
Allergies	Plastic bags
Suffocation	Matches
	Ornaments
	Badly arranged furniture
	Stairs

ACTIVITY 2

Opposite is a plan of a garden. Mark on it where you think there could be possible health hazards.

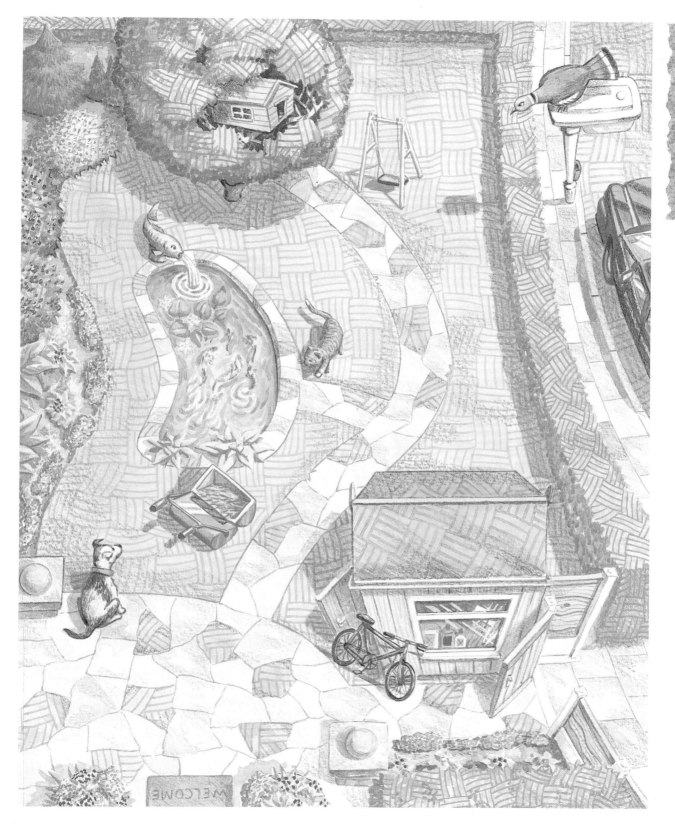

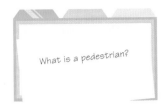

What is a pedestrian?

Hazards on the road

We all use the road at one time or another as pedestrian, cyclist, driver, or passenger.

Pedestrians

Pedestrians face dangers

- **on the pavement**, where uneven surfaces may trip them, shops' goods may overflow on to the pavement, or workmen may have left repairs unguarded
- **on the road** where they can be knocked over by traffic
- **in narrow lanes** where it may be hard for traffic to see them.

Cyclists

Cyclists have little protection in the event of an accident. Wearing a cycling helmet helps to protect them from head injuries. Children on bikes *feel* very visible, as they themselves can see and hear better than they can in a car. They need to be taught that car drivers find cyclists hard to see, especially viewed directly from the front or back, as they don't take up much room. So cyclists need to use all the aids they can to make sure they are noticed.

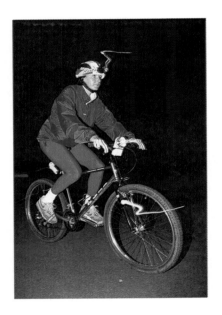

Drivers

A confident driver feels powerful. A warm efficient car protecting you from the rain feels like an extremely safe environment. It is nevertheless a lethal weapon. The driver must be

- able to see clearly
- driving at a safe speed
- in control of the car
- within safe alcohol limits
- alert and not at all sleepy
- concentrating on driving.

Passengers

It is the law that seat belts should always be worn in the front of cars and, if they are fitted, in the rear seats too. It is dangerous for passengers to do anything which affects the driver's concentration, or fiddle about with the car controls. Doors should be locked so that they cannot be opened from the inside by mistake by children or other passengers. The driver's vision should never be blocked by passengers' activities or belongings.

Hazards in social settings

Social settings are those in which people spend their spare time – **recreation** – and those in which they **work**.

NOTE BOOK
Accidents **always** take you by surprise.

unit one

ACTIVITY 3

1 Examine the table below, which outlines ways of helping individuals from different age groups to live within a safe environment.

2 List the main hazards to which adults are exposed.

3 Identify the hazards each of the age groups may be exposed to during different recreational activities.

4 Describe how each of the hazards might affect their health.

5 Describe how the hazards might be reduced.

6 Repeat steps 3 to 5, this time looking at work settings.

7 Make a floor plan of your work room at school or college, marking on it where there are potential safety hazards. [NUM 2.3]

◀▶ Extension opportunity

Find some statistics for accidents in the age groups concerned. Present them in a suitable format. Explain how you checked the validity of the data.

Looking after the safety of different groups of people

Crawlers and toddlers

- Never leave them alone where they could get into a dangerous situation.
- Remember that they can often move faster then you think.
- There is always the first time they begin to climb stairs.
- Look around to make sure everything hazardous is out of reach.
- They will listen to you because they trust you, but they are not able to understand rules.
- Their curiosity gets them into trouble.
- Keep a close eye on them in the garden.
- Teach them safe habits.

Children over 5 years old

- You will not always be with them – they need to develop independence.
- Talk to them often about the dangers they may meet. They should at this age have some understanding of accidents and danger.
- Set them a good example – they will imitate you more readily than they listen to you.
- Let them cook under supervision so they will learn safe habits.
- Encourage them to be tidy.
- Never let them swim alone.
- They are not safe alone on the road. Teach them the Green Cross Code.
- Make sure they learn how to behave safely when travelling in a car – seat belts fastened, not distracting the driver.

Older children

By the time they are old enough to be independent, children need to have learnt safe habits of behaviour.

- Teach them to be in control of their own safety.
- Discuss with them what to do in an emergency.
- Make sure they have proper instruction if they want to take part in dangerous activities.
- Only allow them on the road alone after they are 10 years old, or older, depending on their personalities and abilities.
- Give them road safety training.
- Make sure they wear cycling helmets.
- Encourage them to learn how to maintain cycles in a good, safe condition.
- They must be visible on the road, during the day and after dark.

Adults

- Young adults are more likely to take **calculated risks**. They understand the risks, but expect to 'get away' with dangerous behaviour, that is running across roads, cycling in a risky way, driving a little too fast.
- Older adults tend to be wiser, as their own and their friends' experience may have taught them that dangers and accidents are very real.

Elderly people

- May not recognise their increasing frailty and loss of co-ordination.
- May not see and hear as well as they used to.
- May have thrifty habits which restrict their use of lighting and heating.
- May have homes which need repair and maintenance which have been overlooked.
- Have bones which break more easily.
- May fall because of increasing infirmity or illness.

Hazards in the local environment

The community presents many hazards to people's safety. Schools and offices present their own risks, similar to those in the home yet different, and affected by the greater numbers of people who may be in the building.

The playground

There are similar dangers in the playground to those in the garden, made more complicated by many children playing and competing with each other, although often older children will keep an eye on younger ones.

Railway lines

Railways lines are fascinating to older children because of the very real atmosphere of danger. The trains themselves are scary in their noise and size; the rails are less obviously dangerous, yet can kill by electrocution. The only safe advice to give is STAY AWAY.

Canals

All water is nice to be near. In the country canals are attractive to walk along. In the city they provide a welcome change of environment. But it is hard to climb out of a canal after falling in, as they may be full of rubbish, making it hard to get a foothold. They seldom have shallow edges and are deep all the way across. Safety rules are the same for all water

- hold the hand of those most vulnerable
- teach people to swim
- never trust ice to be thick enough to walk on.

Poisonous plants

Small children, and older people who are confused or have problems understanding the world around them, tend to put things into their mouths, either to explore them out of curiosity, or because they are hungry. Unpleasant tastes, curiously enough, do not discourage them. Berries are tempting and attractive, but all parts of a plant should be regarded as poisonous – flowers, leaves, seeds and berries. It is a good idea to avoid growing plants known to be poisonous where there are vulnerable people.

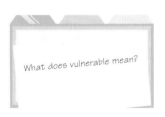

What does vulnerable mean?

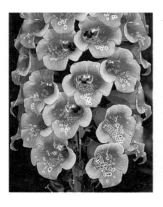
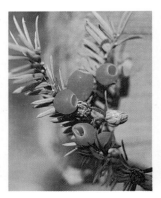
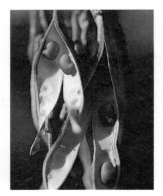
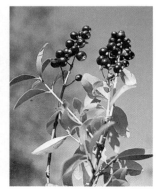

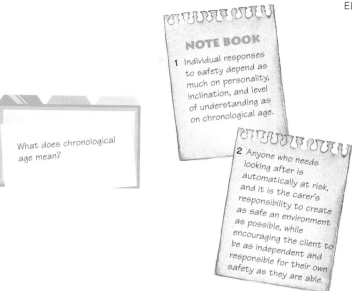

ACTIVITY 4

Collect as many leaflets as you can about safety

1 in the home and garden

2 on the road

3 in social settings (recreation and work)

4 in the local environment.

Put them into the four groups.

What does chronological age mean?

NOTE BOOK

1 Individual responses to safety depend as much on personality, inclination, and level of understanding as on chronological age.

2 Anyone who needs looking after is automatically at risk, and it is the carer's responsibility to create as safe an environment as possible, while encouraging the client to be as independent and responsible for their own safety as they are able.

Performance Criterion 3

Personal Roles and Responsibilities in Dealing with Health Emergencies

You need to know the following steps, 1 to 9, in the order they are mentioned.

1 Assess an emergency

Take a few moments to weigh up the situation calmly; they will be moments well spent.

- Is there any danger to you, others or the casualty?

- What appears to be the immediate situation?

- What clues do the surroundings give you?

2 Maintain your own safety

If you are injured yourself, you will be in no position to help other people.

- Is the situation which caused the original problem under control (fire, gas, flood, electricity)?

- Can you handle it without putting yourself in danger?

- Would it be better for you and the casualty to wait for help?

3 Contact the emergency services

If you have found it necessary to carry out resuscitation the casualty needs to go to hospital and the ambulance service will be needed.

You will always need to call for an ambulance in cases of

- unconsciousness

- difficulty in breathing

- suspected heart attack

- severe bleeding

- serious burns

ACTIVITY 5

Write a short account of how to call the emergency services, and in what order things should be done.

4 Support the casualty physically

This means that you need to be able to look after the casualty's immediate bodily requirements. This means the airway, breathing and circulation. These are covered in pc 5 (see page 62).

5 Support the casualty emotionally

Anyone involved in an accident or emergency suffers some degree of shock, which has emotional as well as physical affects. Whether or not the casualty is conscious, you need to consider their **privacy** and **dignity**.

Privacy means that you

- make sure that clothes are arranged modestly
- avoid exposing the body more than you can help
- prevent the public from prying into other people's misfortune
- discuss personal details with casualties and others in a way which cannot be overheard.

Dignity means that you

- always treat casualties as individuals
- protect them from ridicule if they unavoidably soil or wet themselves
- clean them up as best you can if they are sick
- maintain a sympathetic and reassuring attitude at all times
- ensure that your manner and speech is always courteous, kindly and professional.

6 Work within the limits of your own knowledge and understanding

It would be dangerous to attempt to give treatment that you did not understand or about which you were not certain. Nobody admires those who are arrogant about their abilities. First aid has that name because it is the first help given to those who need it, and after basic life-saving techniques it is wise to pass the casualty over to the emergency services.

7 Transfer the casualty to the emergency services

When an ambulance, the police, or the fire brigade arrive, you will hand over responsibility for the casualty to the personnel of the service concerned. They are trained and equipped to deal with a wide range of situations and will guide you through the process.

8 Describe the event to the emergency services

This involves more than just describing your treatment of any casualties. You need to tell them

- your understanding of what happened

- of any bleeding, vomiting, or unusual behaviour

- of any valuables you may have found and which will need handing over

- if relatives or friends have been informed.

9 Describe to them the support you have already provided

Whenever an incident occurs affecting someone's health, it needs to be reported.

- At home, this is usually informal – we just pass on the information by word of mouth.

- In someone else's home, maybe as a community worker or a baby-sitter, the report ought to be written down.

- In most care settings a recognised accident report is used, and all workers, whether part or full time, paid or voluntary, should make themselves familiar with this as soon as they start work.

- If you are helping out at an accident, jotting this information down and giving it to the right person (ambulance personnel, the patients themselves, or parent or carer) will be useful at the next stage of treatment.

Performance Criterion 4

The Physiological Basis of Basic Life-Saving Techniques for Dealing with Health Emergencies

You need to understand the functioning of the parts of the body most important to keeping a person alive. These are the **circulatory** and **respiratory** systems.

Circulation

Our circulatory system has that name because the blood circulates round the body, just as hot water circulates round a central heating system.

In much the same way and for the same reasons, it consists of a pump – the **heart** – and pipes – the **blood vessels**. If it was not for the heart acting as a pump, the blood would just dribble about and its vital nutrients would never get very far. In **resuscitation** we are most concerned with the **oxygen** dissolved in the blood. If a fresh supply is not carried to the brain regularly, its cells die, and recovery of the casualty may not be complete.

The heart is made of solid muscle, and during life its only resting time is between beats. It is about the size of the owner's fist. As it contracts, waves of pressure pass down the blood vessels leading away from it, which are called **arteries**, and can be felt at our own **pulse points**. The biggest pulse point, carrying the pulse of the large **carotid** artery carrying blood to the head, is in the neck, just behind the voice box. It is called the **carotid pulse** and this is the one which is most important during life-saving procedures.

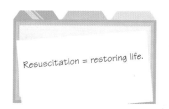

Resuscitation = restoring life.

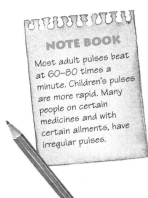

NOTE BOOK

Most adult pulses beat at 60–80 times a minute. Children's pulses are more rapid. Many people on certain medicines and with certain ailments, have irregular pulses.

Like tree branches, the arteries grow smaller and smaller as they go further away from the body; the thinnest blood vessels are called **capillaries**, and through their thin walls oxygen passes to the body tissues and is exchanged for **carbon dioxide**, a waste gas that the body needs to get rid of.

The capillaries which return blood to the heart grow thicker, joining together to form **veins**. Veins carry the blood, now short of oxygen, back to the heart for a final burst of pressure to help the blood to the lungs. In the lungs the carbon dioxide is breathed out, oxygen is breathed in, and the now oxygenated blood travels to the heart for transport round the body.

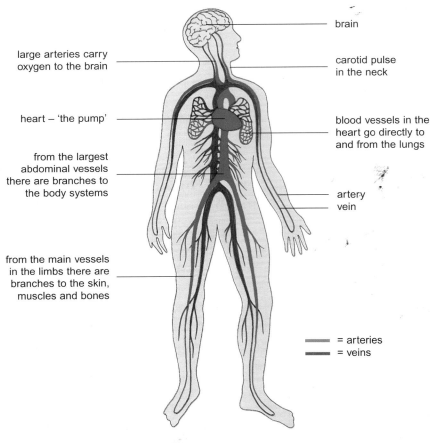

large arteries carry oxygen to the brain

heart – 'the pump'

from the largest abdominal vessels there are branches to the body systems

from the main vessels in the limbs there are branches to the skin, muscles and bones

brain

carotid pulse in the neck

blood vessels in the heart go directly to and from the lungs

artery
vein

= arteries
= veins

How the blood circulates round the body

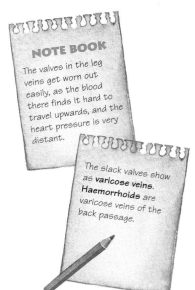

NOTE BOOK

The valves in the leg veins get worn out easily, as the blood there finds it hard to travel upwards, and the heart pressure is very distant.

The slack valves show as **varicose veins**. **Haemorrhoids** are varicose veins of the back passage.

The arteries have thick, muscular walls, and the blood pulses through them. Blood in the veins is more sluggish and the veins have thinner walls, containing valves, to stop the blood flowing backwards.

If the skin is cut the blood coming into contact with air **clots**. This means that it turns into a jelly-like blob, which then solidifies and hardens to stop bleeding from the cut.

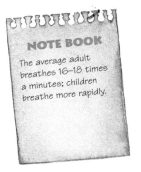

NOTE BOOK

The average adult breathes 16–18 times a minutes; children breathe more rapidly.

unit one

Breathing

Respiration is the proper name for breathing. Oxygen is taken into the **lungs**, where it passes into the blood to be carried round the body via the heart, in the arteries. Carbon dioxide travels back to the lungs in the veins, again via the heart, and is breathed out.

Breathing is stimulated by the amount of carbon dioxide in the blood, which triggers a tiny centre in the brain which determines how often and how deeply we breathe. Thus in mouth to mouth resuscitation, the first aider's breath, rich in its own carbon dioxide, is an extra reminder to the casualty's brain that breathing should start again.

In breathing, the ribs expand, and the **diaphragm** – a sheet of muscle as tight as an open umbrella – is pulled down. This expands the chest cavity and air is sucked in through the nose or mouth into the lungs. When the diaphragm relaxes, the air passes back out.

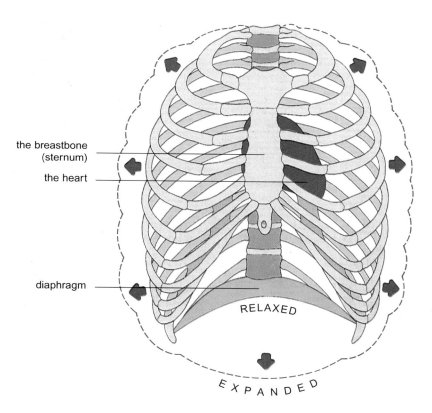

the breastbone
(sternum)

the heart

diaphragm

RELAXED

EXPANDED

The chest expanded and relaxed. The dotted line represents the ribs expanded and the diaphragm pulled down.

Performance Criterion 5

Basic Life-Saving Techniques in Simulated Health Emergencies

After studying this performance criterion you will be able to demonstrate the most important actions for saving life, either in role play or on a resuscitation model.

The first four minutes of someone having an accident or becoming ill are crucial. There is an easy way to remember the sequence of events to follow at this important time, when it would be so easy to panic.

'**Assess**' has already been discussed.

'**Airway**' is explained next.

'**Breathing**' is discussed on page 64.

'**Circulation**' follows on page 65.

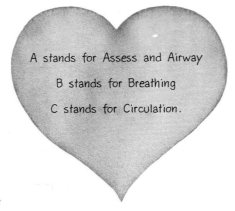

A stands for Assess and Airway

B stands for Breathing

C stands for Circulation.

It's as easy as ABC

ACTIVITY 6

1 Work out what sort of things might block the airway. Think about obstructions that might be

- inhaled
- swallowed
- produced by the casualty.

2 Write them down under the three headings.

Opening and maintaining airways

The airway is the entry to the body for oxygen. Without oxygen the brain cannot function and will become damaged. If you come across an unconscious person who appears not to be breathing, the first thing you do is open the airway in the hope that this simple action will help breathing to start again.

The obvious thing to do is to check for obstructions and remove them. You do this by gently searching the mouth with your bent finger; if you poke about carelessly your fingernail could scratch the throat and cause swelling which would make matters worse. Put a handkerchief round your finger if you have no disposable gloves with you.

Tilting the head keeps the unblocked airway open and this is done by performing a **head tilt**. The **tongue** is a big muscle. Usually, when we are conscious, it is kept busy when we talk and swallow. When we are asleep or unconscious it relaxes, and can flop back, closing the throat and airway. It is attached to the lower jaw and raising this brings the tongue forward clearing the airway. This is called a **chin lift**.

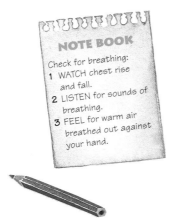

NOTE BOOK

Check for breathing:
1 WATCH chest rise and fall.
2 LISTEN for sounds of breathing.
3 FEEL for warm air breathed out against your hand.

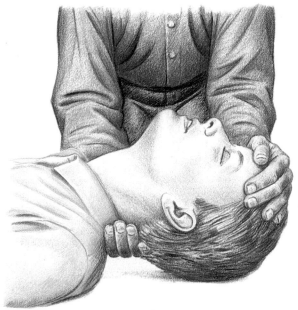

a head tilt,

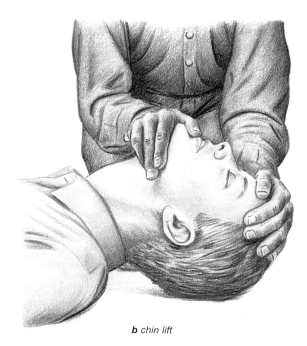

b chin lift

ACTIVITY 7

(You can perform this either on a partner or on a resuscitation model.)

a head tilt

Put the palm of your hand on to the 'casualty's' forehead and gently tilt the head back as far as possible, steadying the neck with the other hand.

b chin lift

Place the fingers of one hand under the bony part of the 'casualty's' chin and pull it upwards and forwards, tilting the head gently backwards with the palm of the other hand.

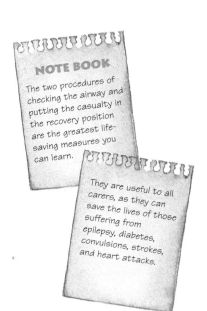

NOTE BOOK

The two procedures of checking the airway and putting the casualty in the recovery position are the greatest life-saving measures you can learn.

They are useful to all carers, as they can save the lives of those suffering from epilepsy, diabetes, convulsions, strokes, and heart attacks.

The recovery position

When turning someone into the recovery position, your aim is to

- move them as little as possible
- keep the head, neck and trunk in as straight a line as possible
- make sure the final position allows fluid to drain out of the mouth instead of spilling back into the lungs
- reduce the chance of the tongue falling back against the throat
- make sure the final position is stable, and the casualty cannot roll.

This is easier to do than to read about, so make sure you ask an experienced first aider to demonstrate.

Helpful hints

- It is easier to remember everything if you start at the head and work downwards.
- Heavy legs are easiest lifted by their clothing.
- If you are wearing a skirt, tuck it under you as it may get trapped when the casualty's weight rolls against you.
- Adjust the casualty in what looks like a comfortable position, as if asleep.
- Be aware that many people are sick as they regain consciousness and fight to clear the airway, so be prepared to move away if the need arises.

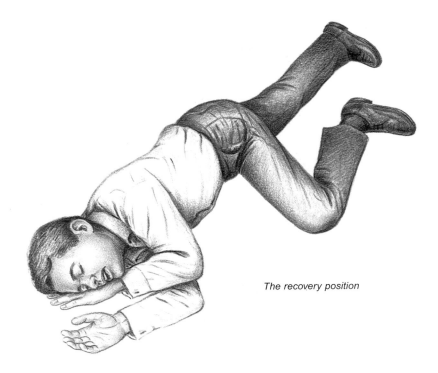

The recovery position

ACTIVITY 8

(You can perform this on a partner.)

The recovery position

Place a partner in the recovery position and have a table like this completed by your assessor to record your competence.

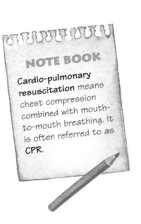

NOTE BOOK

Cardio-pulmonary resuscitation means chest compression combined with mouth-to-mouth breathing. It is often referred to as CPR.

---

1 Kneel, turn casualty's head towards you, tilting it back with the jaw in the open airway position. ☐

2 Place casualty's nearer arm at right angles. ☐

3 Bring far arm over chest tucking hand palm down under casualty' cheek. ☐

4 Cross far leg over near leg. ☐

5 Holding at shoulder and hip, roll casualty towards you. ☐

6 Support casualty, bend upper leg at hip and knee, thigh well up towards chest. ☐

7 Tilt casualty's head back in open airway position. ☐

8 Look at casualty carefully to assess comfort. ☐

Recovery position competence chart

Cardio-pulmonary resuscitation

(You must NEVER perform this on a partner. Practise ONLY on a resuscitation model.)

Breathing

If, when you have cleared the airway, there is still no breathing, you will need to breathe for the casualty. The face will have turned a bluish grey colour.

Helping the casualty to breathe

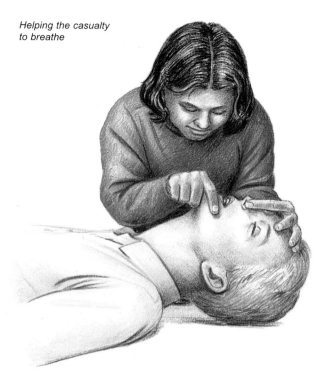

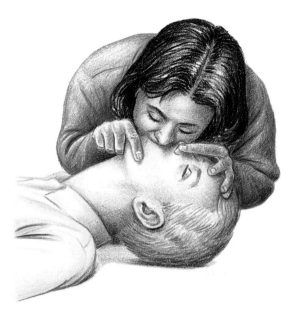

1 *With the casualty flat on the back, keep the airway open and close the nose by pinching it between your finger and thumb. Pull the chin forward and at the same time open the mouth wide.*

2 *Take a deep breath and seal your mouth around the casualty's — you have to open your mouth really wide to be effective.*

3 *Now blow firmly into the mouth. If you can hear or feel air escaping around your mouth you have not got a good enough seal. If the air does not go in, you have not opened the airway enough. Adjust and try again.*

The figure above demonstrates how to breathe for the casualty. You should see the chest rise when you breathe air in, and fall when you take your mouth away. Repeat this about 15 times a minute. The rate and the amount of air you give will vary according to the size of the casualty. With babies or children with small faces you cover the mouth and nose both at once; in cases of mouth injury you can give artificial ventilation through the nose alone while you cover the mouth firmly. You give babies only the amount of air you can hold in your checks, as their lungs are so tiny. You will need to discuss this further with a qualified first aider.

Circulation

If you cannot feel a pulse at the carotid artery in the neck, then the heart has stopped and you must start chest compression. This means that you will be acting as a pump to squeeze blood from the heart into the circulation. The only safe place to do this is over the breast bone. The casualty must be lying flat on the back and it is easier on the floor although it can be performed on a bed. You can straighten the body by pulling firmly down by the ankles.

With children it will be sufficient to give light pressure with one hand only; with babies use only two fingers. As with mouth-to-mouth resuscitation, you will need to discuss this with a qualified first aider.

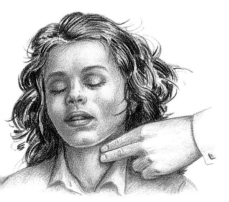

Taking the carotid pulse

Chest compression

1 Kneeling beside the casualty, feel the bottom of the breastbone – practise on yourself. Then measure two finger widths from the bottom and place the heel of one hand above this point.

2 Lock the other hand on top, then with straight arms, compress the chest for about 4–5 centimetres. Adjust this according to the size and weight of the casualty.

3 Pump about 80 times a minute. This is a bit more than one a second and you need to practise the rate until it becomes second nature.

0
1
2
3
4
5

This is 4–5 centimetres

ACTIVITY 9

1 Find your own carotid pulse and that of a partner.

2 Carry out cardio-pulmonary resuscitation on a resuscitation model and have the following table completed by your assessor to record your competence.

Resuscitation competence chart

1 Provide a clear airway within 15 seconds

2 Take a deep breath.

3 Pinch casualty's nostrils.

4 Seal lips around mouth.

5 Blow into lungs until chest rises to maximum expansion.

6 Remove mouth. Watch chest totally deflate.

7 Give further inflation.

8 Check casualty's neck pulse.

9 Hands correctly placed over breastbone with fingers interlocked.

10 Arms straight and vertical press breastbone down 40–50mm to produce carotid pulse.

11 15 chest compressions, at the rate of 80 per minute, followed by two deep inflations.

12 Check neck pulse.

13 Repeat 11 until told that heart and breathing have resumed.

14 If the casualty is neither breathing nor has a heart beat, then you must keep up the pattern of 2 breaths and 15 compressions, repeating this 4 times a minute.

REMINDER

It is important that you never practise these procedures on a living person, as you will interfere dangerously with their body systems.

Controlling haemorrhage

Haemorrhage means bleeding and it can be **external** or **internal**. It can range from a simple graze to a nose bleed, or large blood loss after a serious road accident.

Adults of an average weight have about six litres of blood, and in cases of haemorrhage the amount of blood left in the body goes down. If bleeding continues, or is severe, the body loses its supply of oxygen and important substances and the patient loses consciousness.

Haemorrhage means bleeding and it can be **internal** or **external**.

Internal bleeding does not always show and needs urgent medical attention. If it is inside the skull it can cause pressure on the brain. If it is within the brain the patient suffers a stroke. Fractures can cause bleeding under the skin which appears as bruises. Bleeding within the abdomen may not be diagnosed until the patient becomes quite ill.

External bleeding may be stopped by a first aider. It involves two basic techniques:

1 raising the injured part above the casualty's heart level; and

2 applying pressure.

Squeezing the edges of a wound together allows the blood to start clotting. *This may take as long as a quarter of an hour.* If you cannot press directly on to the injury, you need to press on to the nearest place where an artery passes over a bone. This is called a **pressure point**, and you will recognise it because there will be a pulse there.

When the bleeding seems to have stopped, place a pad over the injury and bandage it firmly in place. Handkerchiefs and scarfs make good first aid alternatives. If blood seeps through this dressing, bind another on top of it, as removing the first may make the bleeding start again.

ACTIVITY 10

1 Find your own pressure points

  a under your arm, where your sleeve seam would run into the arm hole

  b in your leg, halfway down the groin.

2 Draw a diagram to illustrate where you found your pulse/pressure points. [COMM 2.3]

unit one

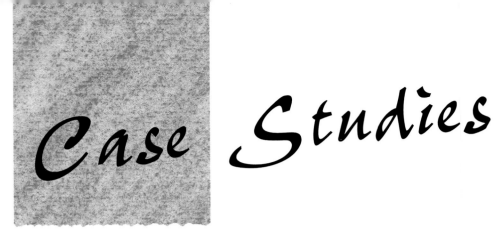

Case Studies

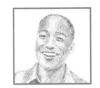

Read the following case studies, and decide which of the alternatives offered would be the best course of action. Use the ABC routine to guide you.

Discuss your decisions in a group.

Case study 1   The Thatched Cottage

George is having a bad morning. He has felt 'peculiar' since he woke up, and needed help with washing, which is unusual. Mark takes him up a coffee and finds him lying on the floor, fully conscious, but still feeling unwell. Should Mark

  a place him in the recovery position and call Dora

  b put him back into bed in his pyjamas

  c leave him where he is and go for help?

Case study 2   Hill Hall

One of the children has epileptic seizures from time to time. At lunchtime she falls from her chair and by the time Ann and Molly get to her she is unconscious, but breathing noisily. Should they

  a check her pulse and prop her up

  b open her airway and put her in the recovery position

  c begin cardiac massage immediately?

Case study 3   Down Way School

It is playtime. Because it has been raining and the grass is wet, the children are not allowed on the field and are playing on the hard area. Several are on the play structures, there is a small quarrel, and Aziz falls off. Isabel is first on the scene. He is unconscious, does not appear to be breathing but his neck pulse is beating. Should she

  a open his airway, give some deep breaths of mouth-to-mouth resuscitation and send a responsible child for help

  b open his airway, begin chest compression and call for help

  c put him in the recovery position and run for the school first aider?

Discussing the incident later, Jalwinder says how impressed she was to see Isabel acting so competently, and how she would like to know what to do if a similar incident should occur.

You are going to work out Isabel's response to Jalwinder.

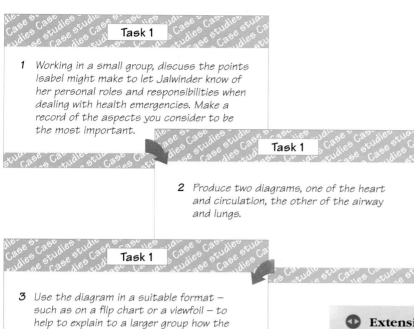

Task 1

1 Working in a small group, discuss the points Isabel might make to let Jalwinder know of her personal roles and responsibilities when dealing with health emergencies. Make a record of the aspects you consider to be the most important.

Task 1

2 Produce two diagrams, one of the heart and circulation, the other of the airway and lungs.

Task 1

3 Use the diagram in a suitable format – such as on a flip chart or a viewfoil – to help to explain to a larger group how the heart and lungs play a crucial part in cardio-pulmonary resuscitation.

Extension opportunity

Bearing in mind that Kevin has asthma, what have you learnt from this element that could be relevant to his state of health?

Case study 4   Netherfield Community Care

Freda is a young adult who lives alone in a small flat. She moves about with difficulty, using a stick or holding on to the furniture. She manages most of her own shopping. Mikhail encourages her to be independent, but Debbie worries about her safety as the flat is very cluttered and is on the second floor.

Task 2

1 Make a plan of your imagined layout of Freda's flat.
2 Mark where there could be a danger from accidents.

Task 2

3 State how Debbie could recommend Freda to reorganise things to make the flat safer.
4 Briefly discuss what Debbie could do if Freda told her to mind her own business.

Multiple Choice Questions

1 Which of the following is the MOST important reason for keeping accurate records after an accident at work? So that

   a *relatives can have a clear picture of what took place*

   b *staff know what treatment has been carried out*

   c *senior staff know that records have been completed*

   d *everyone knows where the patient has gone*

2 When a child falls at school and briefly loses consciousness, which of the following alternatives describes the order in which you would inform people?

   a *the school staff, the parents, the ambulance service*

   b *the parents, the ambulance service, the school staff*

   c *the school first aider, the ambulance service, the parents*

   d *the parents, the school first aider, the headteacher*

3 In what order would you check the casualty's condition

   a *breathing, respiration, pulse*

   b *airway, breathing, pulse*

   c *haemorrhage, pulse, breathing*

   d *attentiveness, bleeding, breathing*

4 How would you first treat a patient with bleeding from the palm of the hand?

   a *lie him or her down and send for an ambulance*

   b *clean the wound with disinfectant and apply a bandage*

   c *apply a sling and take to a casualty department*

   d *squeeze the edges of the wound together and raise the arm*

5 If you are worried about a child you are baby-sitting and ring the parents up to tell them, this is known as

   a *formal reporting*

   b *documented reporting*

   c *informal reporting*

   d *written reporting*

6 Which of the following groups is most at risk of accidents from shop goods displayed on the pavement?

   a *those whose understanding is limited*

   b *those whose vision is limited*

   c *those whose movement is limited*

   d *those whose hearing is limited*

7 Personal roles and responsibilities in emergency situations include

   a *working within own knowledge and understanding*

   b *demonstrating life-saving techniques*

   c *explaining hazards which could cause accidents*

   d *describing the importance of the cardiovascular system*

Summary of Evidence Opportunities and Their Relationship to Performance Criteria

Activities 1, 2, 3 and 4	pcs 1 and 2	**Activity 6, 7, 8, 9 and 10**	pc 5	**Case study 3**	pcs 3 and 4
Activity 5	pc 3			**Case study 4**	pcs 1 and 2

Unit 1 Element 3 Summary of Element Range and Personal Evidence Tracking Record

Element range reference *(tick against left-hand column)*	Description of evidence	Pc and range covered	Portfolio reference number
Pc 1 and pc 2 Hazards			
in the home and garden			
– appliances			
– dangerous substances			
– equipment			
– storage of equipment			
– storage of chemicals			
on the road			
– pedestrian			
– cyclist			
– driver			
– passenger			
in social settings			
– recreation			
– work			
in the local environment			
Individuals			
children			
teenagers			
adults			
elderly people			
Pc 3 Personal roles and responsibilities			
assess emergency			
maintain own safety			
contact emergency services			
support the casualty physically			
support the casualty emotionally			
– protect privacy			
– maintain dignity			
do not exceed own knowledge and understanding			
transfer casualty to emergency services			
describe event to services			
describe to services support provided			

unit one

Unit 1 Element 3 Summary of Element Range and Personal Evidence Tracking Record

Element range reference *(tick against left-hand column)*	Description of evidence	Pc and range covered	Portfolio reference number
Pc 4 Physiological basis of life saving			
circulation			
breathing			
Pc 5 Basic life-saving techniques			
opening and maintaining airways			
placing in the recovery position			
cardio-pulmonary resuscitation			
controlling haemorrhage			

Unit two

UNIT 2

el 2.1	el 2.2	el 2.3
pc 1	pc 1	pc 1
pc 2	pc 2	pc 2
pc 3	pc 3	pc 3
pc 4	pc 4	pc 4
	pc 5	pc 5

unit two

Influences on Health and Well-Being

Elements

2.1 Explore the development of individuals and how they manage change

2.2 Explore the nature of inter-personal relationships and their influence on health and well-being

2.3 Explore the interaction of individuals within society and how they may influence health and well-being

This unit begins by examining personal development and moves on to examine how people interact, first with one another and then within society as a whole.

In the same way as before, the tasks set in this unit develop from each other, to build into a complete record of knowledge to show that you understand fully the influences which combine to affect health and well-being.

Element 2.1

Explore the Development of Individuals and how they Manage Change

Performance Criteria		
pc 1 Describe the main characteristics of development in the different life stages	74
pc 2 Explain the factors which influence an individual's self-concept	84
pc 3 Describe the impact on people of changes caused by major events	88
pc 4 Describe ways in which people manage change caused by major events	90
Summary of evidence opportunities and their relationship to the pcs	95
Summary of element range and personal evidence tracking record	95

Introduction

As we grow and develop during life, we are constantly involved in changes, some of which are quite profound. This element examines these changes; those which are brought about by our physical and emotional development, and those caused by other events. We may or may not have control over these, which in itself will affect how we respond to them.

No two people respond to change in the same way. Our personalities, upbringing and experience all combine to give us a particular view of ourselves, which in turn colours the way in which we cope with life's ups and downs.

Performance Criterion 1

The Main Characteristics of Development in the Different Life Stages

You need to know the usual patterns by which people's bodies and minds develop as they grow from infancy to old age, and how most people become able to manage within society as they mature and develop an understanding of their emotions and relationships. You will be examining physical, intellectual, emotional, and social development. The next diagram illustrates what each of these types of development promote in overall personal development.

EMOTIONAL to promote
confidence
a secure environment
ability to express feelings
ability to cope with anxieties
self-esteem

SOCIAL to promote
independence
awareness of other's needs
communication skills
anti-discriminatory attitudes
sense of social responsibility
comfort with own age group (peers)
good relations with adults
useful role models for others to follow
links between work/school and home
positive ideas about self

PERSONAL
DEVELOPMENT

INTELLECTUAL to promote
creativity
ability to listen
consideration of scientific ideas
observation
language
use of imagination
understanding numbers
enjoyment of art and music
learning through experience
concentration
reasoning

PHYSICAL to promote
bodily control
awareness of space
hand/eye co-ordination
manipulative skills

Physical development

The main stages in our physical development are growth, changes in puberty caused by hormones, maturity, and the ageing process.

Growth in the early stages of life

We develop most quickly during the first five years of life, during which the helpless baby grows into an independent, communicating, responsive child.

The physical skills which develop during infancy are called **motor skills** and depend upon accurate communication between the brain and the muscles. Therefore children who lack such communication will not reach the usual milestones at the same age as most children. However, all *comparative* stages are very general – some children reach them early, others late. Most tend to catch up given time. The diagram below shows motor development comparative stages in the first years of an infant's life

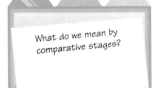

What do we mean by comparative stages?

Motor development

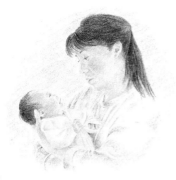

Newborn

Head flops back if unsupported.
Curls forward if put in sitting position.
Lies curled up if put on front.
If held with feet dangling onto a surface makes movements -
the walk reflex.
Grasps anything which is put in hand - grasp reflex.

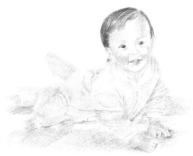

3 months

Begins to control head.
Back starting to straighten if held in sitting position.
Supports weight on bent arms if put on front.
If held upright, legs sag. Walking reflex is lost.
Plays with his or her fingers. Grasp reflex is lost.

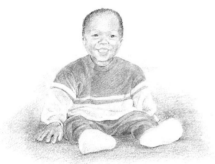

6 months

Can raise head if lying on back.
Sits with hands on floor for support.
Supports weight on straight arms if put on front. Can roll over.
Can take weight on legs if held in standing postion.
Can grasp objects nearby and pass to mouth and other hand.

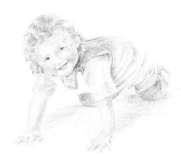

9 months

Has full control of head movements.
Can sit unsupported.
Can crawl clumsily.
Pulls up on furniture to standing and can 'walk' around furniture.
Can pick up small objects.

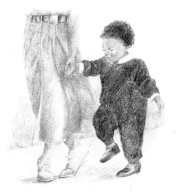

1 year

Can twist and stretch when sitting.
Crawls quickly.
Walks if hand is held to help balance.
Can throw a ball.

15 months walks on own

18 months walks backwards and climbs stairs

2 years kicks a ball
draws

3 years balances on one leg
dresses self

4 years hops

5 years skips

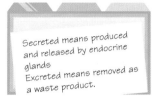

Secreted means produced and released by endocrine glands
Excreted means removed as a waste product.

unit two

Changes in puberty caused by hormones

Children usually continue growing steadily after the age of five until they reach adolescence when growth slows down. It is regulated by messages from their **hormones**.

The hormones are secreted by glands known as **endocrine glands** and are circulated round the body in the blood stream. They are excreted by the kidneys in the urine when they are no longer needed (hence tests for the hormones that indicate pregnancy can be done through a urine test).

All hormone production is regulated by the **pituitary gland** which is found at the base of the brain.

At **puberty** a great surge of hormonal activity causes boys and girls to develop into sexually active men and women. Children grow from infancy in a fairly accepting way, but at adolescence young people are able to be critical of their environment and themselves, and puberty can require quite painful adjustments to be made, especially as there are usually other outside pressures to cope with at the same time.

Puberty in boys occurs when hormones from the pituitary gland stimulate the secretion of male hormones. This causes

- a growth spurt in height
- strengthening of muscles
- more pronounced facial features
- thickening of the vocal cords and enlargement of the Adam's apple
- the voice to 'break'
- appearance of facial and body hair
- development of body odour
- enlargement of the testes, scrotum and penis
- skin and hair to become more oily (acne may develop).

Changes begin internally at around 9 years old, although it is at least three years before any external signs develop. Puberty is generally completed by the age of 18.

Puberty in girls tends to begin and end earlier than in boys. It too depends on messages from the pituitary gland, stimulating the ovaries to secrete hormones. This begins about two years before menstruation.

Although as children girls are usually smaller than boys, their earlier puberty may mean that at the age of 13 they are on average about 2.5cm (1 inch) taller than boys and that they finish their growth spurt before boys begin theirs. Changes at puberty include:

- an increase in height
- appearance of hair under the arms and in the pubic area
- broadening of the hips
- bodily fat being deposited in new places

NOTE BOOK

'Pubic comes from 'puberty', and means to do with the area of sexual organs.

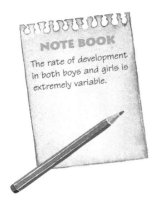

NOTE BOOK

The rate of development in both boys and girls is extremely variable.

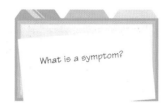

What is a symptom?

- breast development
- **menstruation** (periods starting)
- skin and hair may become more oily and acne may develop.

Maturity

Once through puberty, growth is complete and the body enters the third stage of its life cycle, that of **maturity**. During this period, men and women are able to have children, and bring them up to grow into adults themselves.

In humans this is the longest and most settled time of life, yet before it is over both men and women have to go through another process dictated by their hormone cycle. This is known as the **menopause.**

In women this is more dramatic than in men, and involves the pituitary ceasing to stimulate female hormone production so that menstruation ceases. One side effect of this is that the bones may become brittle, leading to a condition called **osteoporosis**. Other symptoms may include sleeplessness, hot flushes, absent-mindedness and irritability.

These last symptoms may also occur in men as their hormone balance shifts. Bear in mind that around the age of 50 both men and women may be involved in external changes such as job shifts, and it is small wonder that this is often known as the 'mid-life crisis'.

The ageing process

The last stage of physical development is that of old age. Unlike puberty, it is not marked by dramatic changes, but is a gradual process of running down. Described on paper it looks very negative, but at the end of a lifetime of experiences, many people agree that physical age is a case of mind over matter – if you don't mind, then it doesn't matter.

1 Loss of colour in hair.

2 The eyes focus less well. Hearing may become impaired. Taste, smell and touch are less acute. The sense of balance may become affected.

3 Weakened blood capillaries means the skin bruises more easily and red patches may appear under the skin.

4 Breathing is less efficient as the lungs lose elasticity.

6 Arteries thicken inside, so blood circulates less freely. This reduces the oxygen supply and leads to sensitivity to the cold and a raised blood pressure.

7 The brain shrinks, affecting short-term memory. Nerves react more slowly, and responses are slower.

8 Skin loses its elasticity and forms sags and wrinkles.

9 Height loss as bones move closer together. Joints stiffen and enlarge. Muscles lose tone and size. Bones grow more brittle.

10 Digestive organs shrink, so meals need to be smaller.

11 The kidneys and bladder are less efficient.

Physical Effects Of Ageing

The rate of ageing and the extent of physical change involved vary widely between individuals. The table on p.78 describes the physical effects that ageing can produce.

Many of the changes occur as the body and its tissues actually shrink and the systems work less effectively.

Intellectual development

There are three aspects of intellectual development to consider: cognition, language, and memory.

Cognition

The word 'cognition' is similar to 'recognition' and this tells us that it is to do with knowing and understanding.

The outline of cognitive development shown in the photographs is a very simple representation, because so many outside influences affect children's growing understanding of the world.

Cognitive Development
Bear in mind that those people who have learning difficulties may not be able to complete a pattern of development such as the one shown on the right, although opportunity should always be offered to extend and stimulate, and assumptions never made that development has ended.

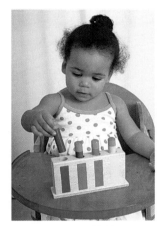

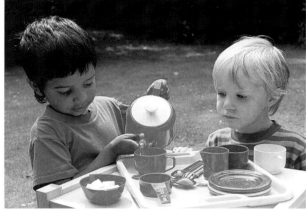

birth to 2 years: child learns directly from his or her actions, rather than by thinking

2–7 years: child lives only in the here and now. Only understands general ideas. Half lives in fantasy land.

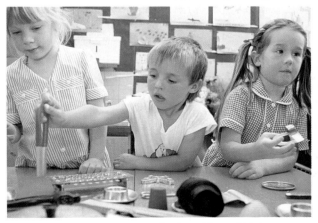

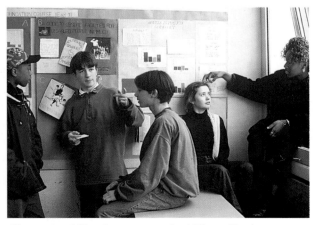

7–12 years: child can think logically about things which have been experienced

12 years to adulthood: can reason about things without experiencing them

unit two

79

Learning

It is tempting to analyse only how *children* learn, forgetting that all of us continue learning throughout our lives, in more or less the same way.

Language development

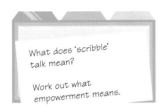

What does 'scribble' talk mean?

Work out what empowerment means.

Development of language depends on effective learning. It takes practice – listening, speaking, responding. Babies speak in 'scribble' talk, then as they develop, become more skilled at forming words. The number of words we know increases as we talk and listen and read throughout life. Language is a tool to clear thought and good communication. All learners, children, young and old, able-bodied or disabled, need time, patience and clear sounds to copy so that as many words as possible can be remembered and used properly.

Language is a key to empowerment for all, including people with no speech, people with hearing impairment, and people who learn slowly.

Infants soon respond to their names and those of their family and toys, and smile when they say these names. They babble to themselves and talk to things as well as people.

ACTIVITY 1

1 Write down ten things you learnt before you were five.

2 Then ten things you have learnt during the last six months.

3 Against them write how you learnt them, from the following list:
   - enthusiasm
   - copying
   - making mistakes
   - encouragement
   - practice
   - you wanted to improve
   - praise
   - useful feedback on progress
   - having ideas
   - success being necessary
   - from a book
   - one thing leading to another
   - guessing

4 Are the learning methods different for the two lists in 1 and 2? If so, why could this be?

5 Record your conclusions in an appropriate and imaginative way.

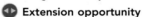 **Extension opportunity**

Link your conclusions to the four stages of your own cognitive development, as outlined in the photographs on page 79.

Memory

Children learn to remember things for longer as they grow older and are encouraged to repeat sounds and experiences. Later they respond to pictures and then to letters and words.

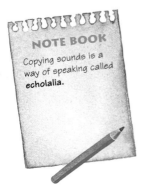

NOTE BOOK

Copying sounds is a way of speaking called **echolalia.**

People with mental health problems make wrong connections with the clues the world gives to them. They may not recognise objects for what they are, but instead may see them as threatening or harmful. No amount of reasoning will convince them that they are misinterpreting what they see.

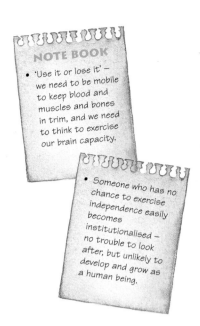

As we grow older, there is more to forget, so our memories seem to suffer. When we are stressed our concentration slips and we make mistakes. Old people may find it easier to remember their childhood than what happened last week.

Emotional development

Good emotional development is encouraged by bonding with others, developing independence and self-confidence.

Bonding

Sound emotional development depends on an individual forming close affection for other people. In infancy this is known as bonding, and begins when a baby is cuddled closely. This means that the main carer is involved, usually the mother, before the circle of affection expands.

When people have learning difficulties, this simple form of bonding may extend beyond childhood. With others, it grows into love and liking for others. When bonding does not occur within the early weeks of life, children can grow up finding it difficult to give or receive affection.

The signs of bonding extend into adult life, and include wanting to touch each other, long eye contact, and response to voice.

Independence

If a person is secure in a loving framework, independence can develop. It begins slowly, in the same way as walking skills do, with practice, encouragement and approval. Small children dare to venture away from their parents until as adolescents they are truly separate people, held to the family only by the invisible links forged during infancy.

All carers should aim to allow those they work with to remain themselves, involved as much as possible in their own care. The balance in this aspect of our lifestyles is especially delicate, as all independence carries a degree of risk. Some carers use this as an excuse to pamper clients, which some of them enjoy, but which is disempowering as it means that the carer is in charge of another person's life. It is physically as well as emotionally damaging, as the body that doesn't move about deteriorates. A person who is independent is one who is able to be free from the control of others.

Emotional security and social ease

A basic human need is to be loved and valued. It is normal for everyone to feel unwanted at some time, but some people feel unwanted most of the time. This can be demonstrated in many ways, such as unacceptable behaviour, withdrawal or seeking attention. This is often easier for the individual than discussing the matter openly, either because people feel reluctant to express their feelings or because they have no language to describe how they feel.

The Balance Of Independence

INDEPENDENCE

- walking alone
- managing money
- making choices
- looking after oneself
- going one's own pace
- using all available help and aids to enable home living

RISK

- falling
- getting into debt
- making mistakes
- not maintaining good health
- taking a long time
- isolation from the community

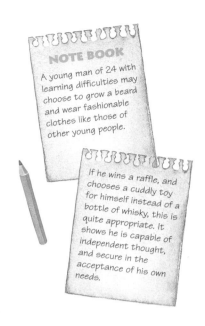

NOTE BOOK

A young man of 24 with learning difficulties may choose to grow a beard and wear fashionable clothes like those of other young people.

If he wins a raffle, and chooses a cuddly toy for himself instead of a bottle of whisky, this is quite appropriate. It shows he is capable of independent thought, and secure in the acceptance of his own needs.

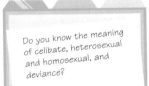

Do you know the meaning of celibate, heterosexual and homosexual, and deviance?

Those who do not live in a family group may well gain their emotional security from their friends and workmates. People of the same age or status as each other are called **peers**. It is inappropriate for children of four, for example, to feel comfortable only in the company of people of their grandparents' age. They need to be able to get on with other young children. People with disabilities need to have the chance to mix with able-bodied friends. This process is called **normalisation**, which means giving everybody access to different styles of living so that they can exercise choice about their lifestyle to the best of their ability.

Personal sexuality is a source of anxiety to some. It is not only concerned with love and acceptance, but also with basic human instincts that can be hard to control. Some people need help in handling sexual urges, and education about the need for responsibility and discretion.

There is the same variety of sexuality among clients as there is among carers. Both groups will include those who choose to remain celibate, both hetero- and homosexual people, and those who have sexual deviances which are not generally accepted in society.

Adolescence, maturity, mid-life, and old age all bring concerns about sexuality which may need to be confronted and resolved. Sexual counselling is a refined skill, and specialist practitioners should be recommended when the need arises.

Self-confidence

With successful independence comes self-confidence, but it is normal for everyone to feel shy and unsure at times, however old or mature they may appear to be. But self-confidence is unattainable without a sound basis of love and security laid down in childhood.

Social development

Co-operation and relationships

Babies are at first completely self-centred. Gradually they begin to realise that other people exist, and so their social development begins. The family is the first group of people of which they become aware, but still they think first of themselves. Then they begin to test the family, in order to discover the limits of the boundaries of their expected behaviour.

Social development is shown by the progressive stages in which children play, and this may be reflected in the way that adults react when they are joining groups with which they are not familiar:

- solitary play – playing alone

- parallel play – playing next to others but not communicating

- looking-on play – watching without joining in

- joining-in play – doing the same thing as everyone else

- co-operative play – belonging to the group and sharing activities.

The pictures below illustrate the pattern of social development in children between 6 months old and 7 years old.

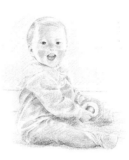

6 months: smiles, attracts attention, makes noises

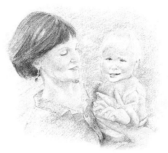

9 months: sees those outside the family as strangers and needs reassuring often

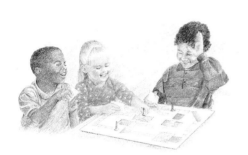

5–7 years: plays co-operatively and understands that rules are necessary

Social Development

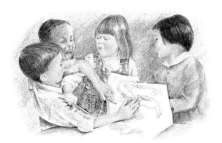

4 years: needs the company of other children but may quarrel with them frequently

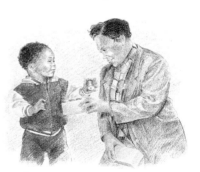

1 year: begins to do as he or she is told, begins to 'help'

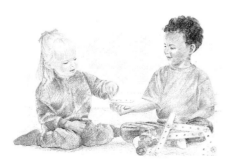

3 years: understands sharing

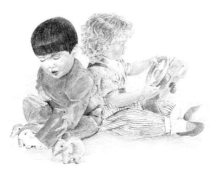

2 years: plays in a group of children, but very selfishly

unit two

83

Performance Criterion 2

Factors Influencing Self-Concept

We all have an idea of who we really are, how we would like to appear to the outside world, and what we would change if we could. It is important to understand the reasons for this opinion of ourselves.

Self-concept means the way in which we see ourselves, and it is very much affected by how other people see us. We view ourselves in the mirror of other people's opinions, and the reflection we see depends on many aspects of our background, experience and personality. Factors influencing self-concept include:

- education
- gender
- emotional maturity
- sexual maturity
- appearance
- age
- culture
- relationships
- work.

Education

Education is not to be confused with the intellectual development examined in the first performance criterion. It is to do with our upbringing and our schooling, and how much this has done to enrich our self-confidence and self-esteem.

ACTIVITY 2

1 Think about the following statements:

a Feminism has ceased to be a new phenomenon in the United Kingdom and some maintain that women have overtaken men in matters of gender equality.

b As single mothers bring up children successfully, some of those children may begin to question the need for constant fathering.

c Male unemployed graduates outnumber female unemployed graduates.

d Females begin to be better qualified than men. However, more men than women hold the most powerful jobs.

2 Working in a small group, decide some possible results of the four situations 1 a-d and how they might affect individuals during their

a infancy and childhood

b adolescence

c early adulthood

d mid-life

e old age.

3 Share your group's opinions with your tutor group, and record those which the majority considers to be significant.

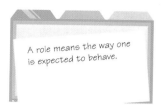

A role means the way one is expected to behave.

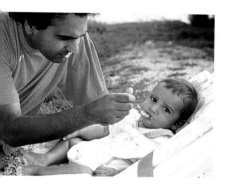

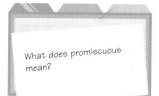

NOTE BOOK

Young children are aware at a very early age whether they are girls or boys.

Many men are insisting that they become more involved with their children.

What does promiscuous mean?

Gender

Gender means sex; male or female. All around us there are images of how men and women are supposed to behave. These images are called 'stereotypes', and they can be very unhelpful to an individual trying to etablish their own identity. Traditionally women were stereotyped as housewives, and men as money earners, but these roles are no longer relevant to many people's lives.

This is an important factor in an individual's self-concept; without confidence in your gender role it is hard to know quite who you are, and our perception of ourselves can depend to a large extent on what we think is other people's opinion of us.

Emotional maturity

We all need to love and be loved. Without the bonding experience described earlier, it is difficult for adults to form the normal, accepting friendships which indicate emotional maturity. Those with low self-esteem find it hard to see anything reflected off those around them which shows there to be anything lovable in themselves.

In our society, which promotes the image of the ideal body, it can be especially easy for people who have disfigurements or deformities to see themselves as ugly. If, during their education and upbringing, they are constantly respected as individuals worthy of receiving love, they are more likely to develop into emotionally mature adults.

Conversely, some adults who are emotionally immature feel themselves to be ugly when they are not. This is quite common during growing up. Most people grow out of it as they see themselves to be accepted as normal people by their friends.

Sexual maturity

After puberty, a person is sexually mature. It is a physical state brought about, as we have seen, by hormonal changes. During the process many emotional changes also take place, and a person's self-concept often becomes confused, but this is usually only temporary. With sexual maturity comes the ability to be sexually active. If emotional maturity lags behind, this can result in sexual behaviour which is promiscuous or inappropriate.

People with learning difficulties may be sexually mature, yet not have the social or emotional maturity to know when, where, or how it is acceptable to have sexual relationships. People with psychiatric illnesses may be unable to control their sexual urges, despite being sexually mature.

These complications make sexual maturity a complex factor in a person's self-concept.

Appearance

We have examined how we 'see' ourselves and how we may think others 'see' us, but have been thinking about ideas rather than what is simply seen with the eyes. Now we come to actual appearance; physical characteristics, clothing, and body language. We all have confused images when we think of our physical characteristics, when all most people see is a perfectly normal person.

So we cover our confusion with clothes, either different from everyone else's if we want to make a point, or as like everyone else's as possible if we want people to associate us with a particular group.

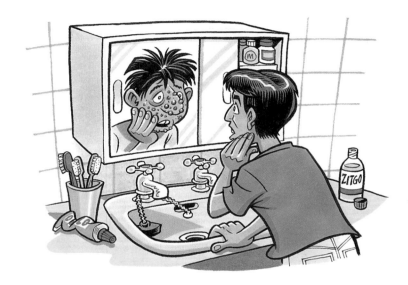

ACTIVITY 3

1 What image might these people be hoping to project to those who see them?

2 Are they trying to be different from or the same as others in their group?

3 Conduct two surveys among a cross-section of males and females to see which clothes they prefer to wear.

4 Present the information from your findings in graphical form(s). [NUM 2.1, 2.3]

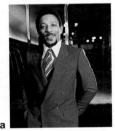
a

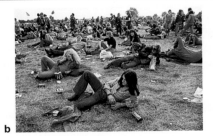
b

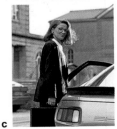
c

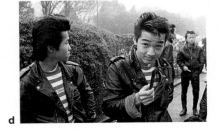
d

ACTIVITY 4

1 Describe how you think **a** a 7 year old girl, **b** a 30 year old woman, **c** an 18 year old man, and **d** a 70 year old woman would behave

   • in a queue at the fish and chip shop

   • on a bus

   • caught in a rain storm.

2 If they behaved in another, very unpredictable way, talk about what this might suggest they thought about themselves and their age.

Age

Society expects people to behave in certain ways according to their age. Use Activity 4 on the left to help you to think about this.

Culture

Our ideas of ourselves are formed by the people who surround us.

‘Little girls should be seen and not heard’

‘Little boys don't cry’

‘Men must work and women must weep’

Sayings like this give us ideals, and when we break away from them we sometimes become stronger in our self-concept and sometimes feel guilty because we have not done what is expected of us.

Different cultures impose different expectations of language, music, literature, religion and lifestyle. Sometimes men are very dominant, and women are subservient – culture and gender combining as factors affecting self-image.

Some examples of cultural expectations are arranged marriages, ‘suitable’ employment, respect for grandparents. The response of our culture to our chosen lifestyle is an important factor in how we feel about ourselves as adults.

Relationships

As we grow up and become independent, our relationships extend beyond from the family. We often adjust our conduct according to the company in trying to gain approval. Behaviour changes subtly as our self-concept shifts when we see ourselves through other people's eyes.

ACTIVITY 5

1 List the people you have met today.

2 Describe your relationship with each of them. Here are some relationships which may fit:
admirer, friend, acquaintance, colleague, sister/brother, member of the public, employee, son/daughter, student, stranger.

3 Describe how your behaviour has changed as you have responded to each person.

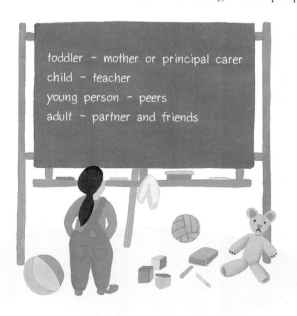

Whom Do We Admire?

Work

'What do you do?' is often the first question you are asked after your name. Many people see themselves mainly in the light of their jobs and when answering, we say: 'I am a nurse', 'I am a footballer', 'I am a classroom assistant', not 'I work as a nurse', 'I work as a footballer', 'I work as a classroom assistant', which shows how much we identify with our jobs. This is a problem when people become unemployed, stay at home to care for someone else, or retire, after seeing their work as a necessary part of their existence.

For people who have never worked, and who may have had many rejections during their search for work, self-esteem can be very low. It is important for the community to reinforce that everybody is precious and important, regardless of their employed status.

Performance Criterion 3

The Impact on People of Changes Caused by Major Events

Sometimes the things that happen to people are expected, sometimes they are a surprise, either enjoyable or unpleasant. Either way, people can react in a variety of ways which you need to know about if you are to respond sympathetically to those you look after, or to understand the effects of life experiences on yourself.

The things that happen to us fall into two main groups; those we expect, which are **predictable**, and those we do not, which are **unpredictable**.

Predictable events

The predictable events in a person's life might include:

- starting school
- starting work
- leaving home
- marriage
- having children
- changing job
- moving home
- retirement.

It is easy to think that these are positive experiences, leading to new possibilities, yet even exciting events cause stress in our lives, especially when we worry that things may not turn out well.

What you felt is shared by everyone confronted by **change**, from a small child starting play-school to a mature adult changing a job, a patient recovering from an operation and about to go home, or a young person with a disability getting a first car which will bring independence and mobility.

ACTIVITY 6

1 Think of some predictable events that have happened to you.

2 What did you feel as they came nearer?

Here is a list to help:

apprehension, uncertainty, loneliness, anxiety, inadequacy, fear of failure, fear of the known, sick, fear of responsibility, fear of looking foolish, nervous, tension.

Present your conclusions using images. Use a computer if you wish.

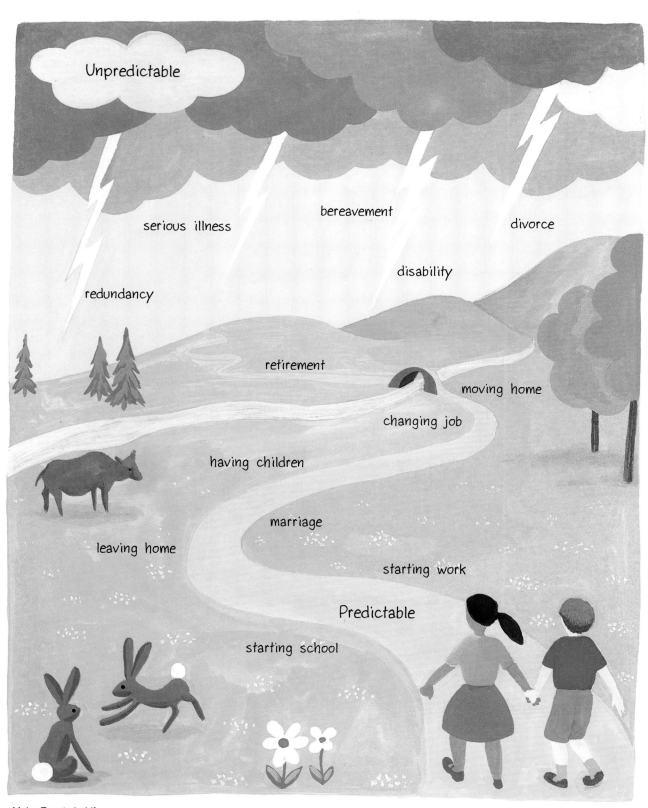

Unpredictable

serious illness

bereavement

divorce

disability

redundancy

retirement

moving home

changing job

having children

marriage

leaving home

starting work

Predictable

starting school

Major Events In Life

Unpredictable events

The unpredictable events in people's lives bring *elements of bereavement*, which means **loss**. The loss may be in the form of redundancy, where a job is lost; serious illness, where health is lost; disability, where ability is lost; divorce or separation, where a relationship is lost; and bereavement, where a person's physical presence is lost through death.

The stages of bereavement have been mapped, and apply broadly to all the unpredictable events listed:

1 Denial and disbelief – 'I don't believe it'.

2 Anger – 'How can this happen to me?'

3 Depression – 'Things will never be the same again'.

4 Despair – 'I can't go on'.

5 Adjustment – 'Life must go on'.

6 Acceptance – 'It's up to me now'.

Individuals react to these unexpected events in different ways, some adjusting more quickly than others. Much depends on the amount of additional stress in their lives at the same time, their personality, and their self-esteem. Examples of possible responses to predictable and unpredictable events are given in the diagram below.

Possible Responses To Events

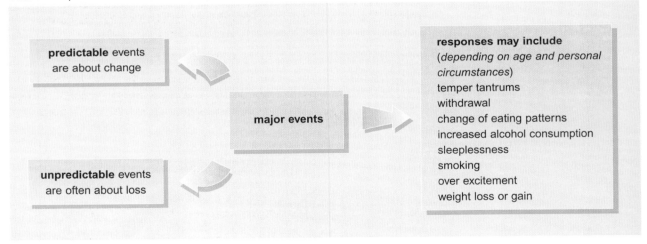

predictable events
are about change

major events

unpredictable events
are often about loss

responses may include
(*depending on age and personal circumstances*)
temper tantrums
withdrawal
change of eating patterns
increased alcohol consumption
sleeplessness
smoking
over excitement
weight loss or gain

Performance Criterion 4

Ways in Which People Manage Change Caused by Major Events

This performance criterion follows on from the last, and examines how people cope with their response to change and what personal support, such as family, social, or professional help, they might use. When important changes occur in life, individuals seek comfort and help in many ways.

Family support

People look for support in the way which is best for themselves and for the situation they find themselves in. Many turn to their families first.

Social support

Social support can come from friends, colleagues and the community in which we live:

- religious leaders
- clubs and social groups
- school or college
- ethnic community groups.

Professional help

Professional help can be general, or specific for certain situations. For example, **medical help** could come from the family doctor, practice nurse, special clinic, pharmacist, community nurse or health visitor, or health centre; **financial help** could come from social security benefits, local authorities, or educational grants.

Some people need convincing that welfare benefits are their right – elderly people sometimes view them as charity. Since in this country we all pay tax either through work or on the things that we buy, everyone in need is entitled to state benefits. They are preferable to private loans and credit schemes (hire purchase) which may grow beyond the borrower's control. **Advisory help** includes

- public services (e.g. Citizens Advice Bureau)
- voluntary organisations with specialist knowledge (e.g. British Red Cross Society, Diabetic Association, Mencap, National Society for Prevention of Cruelty to Children, Alcoholics Anonymous, The Terence Higgins Trust)
- counselling services.

unit two

ACTIVITY 7

1 Read again your list of predictable major events and your reactions to them (see Activity 6).

2 Remind yourself how you were helped to cope with your feelings until you felt able to manage alone.

3 Sort them under the following headings: family, social, professional help.

4 Record the information in a suitable way.

Case Studies

The students at The Thatched Cottage, the health care team in Netherfield, and staff at Down Way School all have to prepare case studies. The first stage is to examine the changes in some of their clients' lives.

You are then going to prepare the first part of the three case studies that Mark, Debbie and Jalwinder are undertaking.

Case study 1 The Thatched Cottage

Rosa is a resident with age-related confusion. She is an identical twin who became deaf in one ear when she was a child. She lives with her husband in a twin room in The Thatched Cottage, having moved from a large rambling house to be nearer her family. Mark is preparing a case study to identify the changes in Rosa's life.

Case study 2 Netherfield Community Care

Debbie becomes interested in Mishka, a widow from Poland living in the town. She speaks little English, but can understand it quite well. Her son was diagnosed as having schizophrenia, and Mishka was devastated when he began to live rough, although things have improved since he came under the care of the health care team. Debbie asks Mikhail to help her ask Mishka if she can use her life experiences for a case study.

Case study 3 Down Way School

Jalwinder would like to prepare a case study about Tim. He came to the school very withdrawn and apparently able to speak only a few words. Six months later he is chatty and settling well. He lives down the road from Jalwinder, and Isabel knows his mother well. Jalwinder has few clues about the changes in Tim's life.

Task 1

1 List the changes which you think might have taken place in each of the three clients' lives.
2 Classify them as predictable or unpredictable.
3 Word process your findings, save on disk and print. **[IT 2.1, 2.2]**

Task 1

Discuss as a group the ethical issues of exploring the private lives of those in care.

Task 1

4 Identify one major event in each classification.
5 How might the clients and/or their families have managed the resulting change?
6 How might the students find out what the changes have been?

Case study 4   Hill Hall

Ann is beginning to come to grips with the emotional stress of working with disabled children, and Molly is keen that she doesn't lose touch with the reality of the average child's development. She asks Ann to do a comparative study of Usha, a Hindu girl with physical and mental disabilities resulting from cerebral palsy, and Ann's sister Lucy, who is the same age and has no disabilities. Ann is to begin by describing the main characteristics of development in the different stages of life, beginning at infancy and ending with old age. Next she is to list the factors which influence an individual's self-concept, keeping it general and not specific to either Usha or Lucy.

Task 2

1 Produce the sort of information which Ann would make under the two headings of 'Development' and 'Self-concept'.

Task 2

2 Make a table which shows the possible links between the factors influencing self-concept and the different stages of development.

You may find the summary of the element range on page 95 helpful.

Multiple Choice Questions

1 Which of the following is a *predictable* major life event?

  a *disability*

  b *having children*

  c *divorce*

  d *illness*

2 Changes at puberty are caused by

  a *diet*

  b *ageing*

  c *hormones*

  d *gender*

3 Education, appearance, maturity and relationships all affect an individual's

  a *self-destruction*

  b *selfishness*

  c *self-analysis*

  d *self-concept*

4 Which *one* of the following is an intellectual characteristic?

  a *independence*

  b *cognition*

  c *gender role*

  d *bereavement*

5 When a mother and baby forge strong emotional links, this is known as

  a *motherhood*

  b *recognition*

  c *bonding*

  d *contact*

6 If the main earner in the family is made redundant, which *one* of the following would be the *most* useful?

  a *counselling by Relate*

  b *consultation with the family's GP*

  c *professional help from the social services*

  d *appointment of an advocate*

7 Which of the following affects a person's physical characteristics?

  a *growth and maturity*

  b *cognition and bonding*

  c *personal relationships and hormones*

  d *puberty and independence*

8 Which of the following phrases *best* describes the impact on a family of the birth of a child with severe physical disabilities?

  a *an acquired disability problem*

  b *problems with intellectual development*

  c *a factor influencing self-concept*

  d *an unpredictable major event in life*

Summary of Evidence Opportunities and Their Relationship to Performance Criteria

Activity 1	pc 1	Case studies 1, 2 and 3	Pcs 3 and 4
Activities 2, 3, 4 and 5	pc 2	Case study 4	Pc 1
Activity 6	pc 3		

Unit 2 element 1 Summary of Element Range and Personal Evidence Tracking Record

Element range reference (tick against left-hand column)	Description of evidence	Pc and range covered	Portfolio reference number
Pc 1 Characteristics of development			
physical – growth			
– changes in puberty caused by hormones			
– reaching maturity			
– the ageing process			
intellectual – cognition			
– language			
– memory			
emotional – bonding			
– independence			
– self-confidence			
social – co-operation			
– relationships			
Stages in life			
infancy to childhood			
adolescence			
early adulthood			
mid-life			
old age			
Pc 2 Factors affecting self-concept			
education			
gender			
emotional maturity			
sexual maturity			
appearance			
age			
culture			
relationships			
work			

unit two

Unit 2 element 1 Summary of Element Range and Personal Evidence Tracking Record

Element range reference (tick against left-hand column)	Description of evidence	Pc and range covered	Portfolio reference number
Pc 3 People			
self			
others – of different gender			
– of different ethnic origin			
Major events			
predictable – starting school			
– starting work			
– leaving home			
– marriage			
– having children			
– changing job			
– moving home			
– retirement			
unpredictable – redundancy			
– serious illness or disability			
– divorce			
– bereavement			
Pc 4 Support in managing change			
family support			
social support			
professional help – medical			
– financial			
– advisory			

Element 2.2

Explore the Nature of Inter-Personal Relationships and their Influence on Health and Well-being

Performance Criteria

pc 1	Describe the relationships formed in the contexts of daily life	97
pc 2	Describe causes of changes in relationships	100
pc 3	Describe reasons why people form relationships	102
pc 4	Explain the role of the family in the development of individuals	104
pc 5	Identify the consequences of breakdown in relationships on health and well-being	105
	Summary of evidence opportunities and their relationship to the pcs	111
	Summary of element range and personal evidence tracking record	111

unit two

Introduction

Having examined how individuals develop and how they manage the expected and unexpected changes in life, we now look at how they relate to one another.

Different kinds of relationships are described and these are looked at to see how they are affected by the changes already studied. Family influences on people's development are explained, and lastly the effects of relationships breaking down are examined.

Performance Criterion 1

The Relationships Formed in the Contexts of Daily Life

In the process of growing up and going about our ordinary daily life, we meet other people. We interact with them and form **relationships**. We hold different sorts of relationship with different people. Those differences are examined in this performance criterion.

There are three main areas in which we interact with others.

The family

Our experiences of other people start within the family. As most of us have families, it is easy to make assumptions about other people's.

You may find that any assumptions you may hold about all families being like your own are far from accurate. Some people have strong

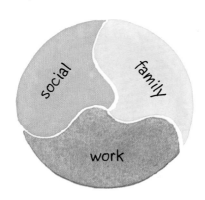

Three areas of interaction

ACTIVITY 1

1 Write down the names of your immediate family (parents, brothers and sisters).

2 Use a drawing software package on a computer to show the relationships there are between family members. (Pets can be very important members of the family, and often strong bonds are formed with them.) **[IT 2.1, 2.2]**

3 Compare the diagram of your own family with other people's.

4 Repeat steps 1, 2 and 3 with your extended family.

(The wider or **extended family** = relatives other than your immediate family such as aunties, uncles, grandparents.)

5 What differences can you see between your diagram and other people's?

◄► **Extension opportunity** Conduct a survey within the group of the different types of relatives existing – e.g. number of uncles, brothers, sisters.

Categorise these relations into age groups to present the information in a more detailed form. **[NUM 2.1, 2.3]**

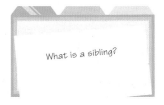

What is a sibling?

family bonds, but few members of the family. Others have several grannies and uncles and step-siblings, and are able to keep only distant contact with them all.

The differences come about because of

- geography – they may or may not live far apart
- family habits – they may or may not meet often
- culture – some cultures have strong traditions of family support
- partnering patterns – divorce and separation are more frequent in some families than others.

Work

People working together often become a mixture of friends and colleagues. This usually happens between individuals who have a similar role in the workplace.

Informal and formal relationships at work

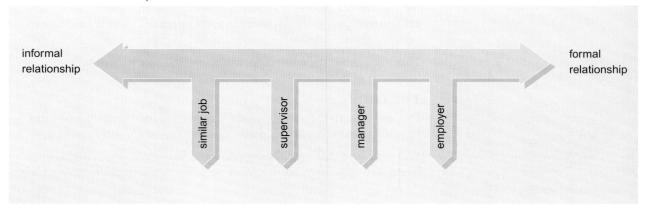

Relationships become more formal with those furthest away from the individual's employed status. The bigger the establishment, the wider the gulf between employer and employee. In smaller establishments, relationships between the individual and 'the boss' are often less formal. Much, of course, depends on the atmosphere of the workplace and the personalities involved.

> Do you know the difference between an employer and an employee?

Social

Any relationships which are not based in either the family or at work are social ones. Whenever two or more people meet, some relationship is inevitably formed. When people know each other well, their relationship is **intimate**. When they hardly know each other, it is a **distant** relationship.

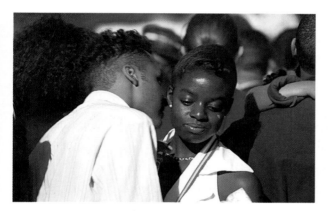

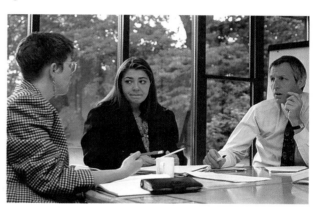

unit two

ACTIVITY 2

1 Whom have you met since this morning? Try to remember everyone.

2 Work out whether your relationship was a family, work or social one.

3 Which were distant and which were intimate relationships?

4 Use a method of recording your findings which will enable you to use percentages and ratio when you describe the different types of relationships. [**NUM 2.2**]

The social group is often the largest of the three, as it includes

- friends
- members of clubs
- recreational groups
- cultural groups
- the immediate community

ACTIVITY 3

1 Explain what is meant by 'the immediate community'.

2 Describe your own.

3 Work out the relationships which exist between you and members of your own immediate community.

4 Record your findings in an appropriate and imaginative way.

> cultural groups = those who share one another's ideas, beliefs and values.

Performance Criterion 2

The Causes of Changes in Relationships

Changes occur as we grow older and develop, and also as expected and unexpected events affect our lives. These changes have been examined in depth in Element 1, pcs 1 and 3. Here it is their impact on our relationships which is explored.

So far we have looked at simple relationships, mainly between two people. If you look back at the diagrams resulting from Activity 1, it is obvious that life is seldom as simple as this. Everybody interacts, affecting everybody else's relationships.

If there is a change in any one relationship everyone else involved feels some effect. This applies especially to relationships within the family.

Stages in life and their effect on relationships

As family members progress from childhood to adolescence, from adulthood to old age, interaction with other members of the family shifts and alters.

No person is ever static. All family members are developing, either quickly (as babies) or slowly (as adults) and if two of them meet a crisis point at the same time, life can become quite difficult for the family as a whole.

Life stage conflicts

		infancy	childhood	adolescence	adulthood	mid-life	old age
		A	B	C	D	E	F
infancy	1						
childhood	2						
adolescence	3						
adulthood	4						
mid-life	5						
old age	6						

ACTIVITY 4

1 Look at the grid in the table oppsite.

2 Describe what might happen in square, E3, A2, and F5 if those concerned were undergoing a major age-related change. Imagine the relationship in terms of

   a a happy outcome

   b a stressful outcome

   c a disastrous outcome.

3 Write an imaginary scenario to explain how this changed relationship between two people might affect others in the family.

event

changes

▽

role

changes

▽

self concept

changes

▽

behaviour

changes

▽

relationship

Major events and their effects on relationships

At the same time as we grow and develop, we have to cope with the change and loss which is part of life's experience. Sometimes as family members change, the altered relationship becomes a crisis in itself, for example

a the arrival of a baby

b a young adult about to become independent is permanently disabled in an accident

c death of parents

d a grandparent has to move in with the family.

The change in relationships is bought about by the change in role of the individuals involved. For the above cases

a a career woman might become a mother

b an adult might become as dependent as a child

c an adult son might feel alternately an orphan and head of the family

d a grandparent might have the physical needs of a baby.

The four points above only describe the effect on one person. Everyone else in the family has to adjust to this new pattern.

When we looked at self-concept in the last element, we saw that we project our self-image on to the world by our behaviour. When we change our role, we sometimes have to adjust our self-concept at the same time, and our behaviour may change.

Our friends and acquaintances themselves constantly change and adjust their roles and self-concepts and may start to treat us differently, and so relationships are affected.

Performance Criterion 3

Reasons why people form relationships

In this performance criterion we see why people strike up friendships and other types of relationships. We enter into relationships for three interlinked reasons; emotional, intellectual, and social.

ACTIVITY 5

1 Using the table below choose one reason from each of the three categories which could lead to a negative or harmful relationship.

2 Describe the possible results on those involved and record the results.

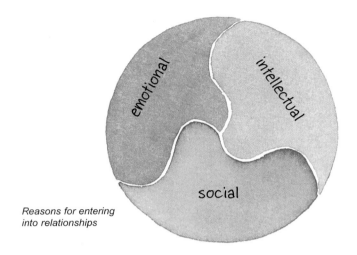

Reasons for entering into relationships

They are linked because as human beings our actions are too complicated to stem from one single cause.

Reasons why people form relationships

EMOTIONAL	INTELLECTUAL	SOCIAL
• a search for identity • comfort • approval • security • the need to belong* • independence* • attraction of opposites* • pressure from peers* • rebellion*	• improvement/stimulus • ambition • independence* • attraction of opposites* • reflection of ideas	• shared interest • conformity • rebellion* • company • pressure from peers* • attraction of opposites* • need to belong*

* Some reasons occur in more than one category, others seem to cancel each other out. This reflects people's individuality.

Nothing has been said so far about quality of relationships. Some of the reasons for forming relationships given in the table above are negative, some of them could even be harmful.

Attraction of similar personalities

We are often attracted to people like ourselves. In our social life we meet others from the same cultural background. Partnerships are often formed between people of a similar level of education. We may make friends with individuals with the same emotional needs as ourselves.

Attraction of opposite personalities

We can all think of unlikely couples who remain apparently happily attracted to each other. However, it is sometimes difficult to understand how and why people who are so different find the relationship rewarding.

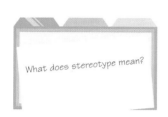

What does stereotype mean?

ACTIVITY 6

Match the personality stereotypes below to their opposite.

quiet	helpless
villain	loser
carer	scatter-brained
winner	admirer
organised	victim
show-off	outward going

unit two

The **emotional** reason for such relationships is that a person showing the opposite characteristics allows us to indulge our secret ideal role.

'I want a wife who reminds me of my mother.' / 'I want a husband I can organise.'

'I want to stay a little girl.' / 'I need a wife I can pamper.'

'I like to feel powerful.' / 'I will look for a husband who will take charge of me.'

Intellectually, we choose someone different from ourselves to help us with the things we find difficult.

'I want to improve my badminton.' / 'I need a badminton partner, but I would still like to win most of the time.'

'I am good at maths but bad at humanities.' / 'I am good at humanities and need help with my maths homework.'

Or we may have a relationship which will make up for our shortcomings in **social** circumstances.

'I am scared to ask girls out, my mate's much better at it than I am.' / 'I'm OK with girls. It makes me look even better if I help him out.'

'I am nervous in busy shops, but want to go to town at the weekend.' / 'I want a friend who enjoys going round the shops on Saturdays.'

You will see that **emotional** undercurrents underlie the **intellectual** and **social** reasons.

Independence

Since independence implies freedom, it seems a strange reason for forming a relationship, as all relationships bring responsibilities and ties. Independent people will select friends who allow them to operate as a free agent, without making too many demands on them, either emotionally or otherwise.

Stimulus

In order to develop our minds and intelligence we all need to be extended, otherwise we stagnate and life becomes boring. This requirement for well-being is the same for those with learning difficulties as it is for everyone else. Fastening a button may extend the abilities of someone with poor eye-hand co-ordination. Splitting an atom extends the scientist.

People may nurture relationships in order to increase their skills, or knowledge, or just to make their life generally more invigorating.

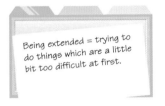

Being extended = trying to do things which are a little bit too difficult at first.

Performance Criterion 4

The Role of The Family in the Development of Individuals

Families, in their raising of children, play a crucial role in the development of individuals. We carry all through our lives the good and the bad things we learnt from our families in childhood.

A family is a group of people of various ages, related by birth, marriage or adoption. It is the basic unit of society.

Society is built up of families

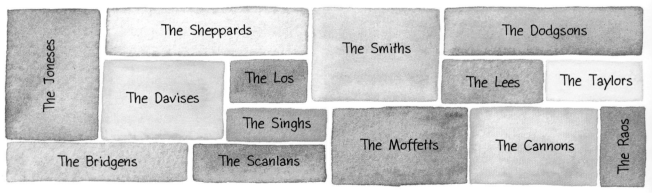

The Joneses · The Sheppards · The Smiths · The Dodgsons · The Davises · The Los · The Lees · The Taylors · The Singhs · The Moffetts · The Cannons · The Raos · The Bridgens · The Scanlans

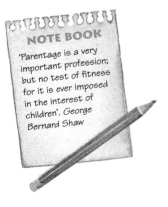

NOTE BOOK

'Parentage is a very important profession; but no test of fitness for it is ever imposed in the interest of children'. *George Bernard Shaw*

Families

In a wider context the family unit could be a father, his children and his girlfriend, or a mother and daughter and her boyfriend, or a couple in a caring loving homosexual relationship who live together.

The three roles of **protection**, **provision** and **support** are most intense when there are children in the family, but they combine throughout family members' lives. Some close families protect, provide and support many members very actively over periods of time. Other

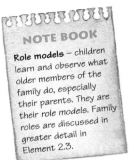

NOTE BOOK

Role models – children learn and observe what older members of the family do, especially their parents. They are their role models. Family roles are discussed in greater detail in Element 2.3.

families move apart and the roles are then taken over by friends or society. Much depends on learnt family behaviour patterns, circumstances, personalities, and cultural expectations.

Children from families where protection, provision and support are absent or incomplete, or parenting is inadequate – in particular when love and affection are missing – do not thrive emotionally or physically and are said to be **deprived**. Such children may grow into adults who have difficulty in forming satisfactory relationships, as they have been unable to develop fully as individuals.

The role of the family

PROTECTION	PROVISION	SUPPORT
• food	• protection (see previous list)	• love and affection
• shelter	• education	• understanding
• warmth	• financial help	• mutual respect
• clothing	• support (see following list)	• sense of belonging
• training in how to be social individuals	• role models	• promoting self-esteem
• immunisation against disease	• advice on problems	• encouraging independence
• providing experiences to increase independence		• helping one another as circumstances change
		• visiting and companionship
		• maintaining family traditions to give a sense of continuity

Performance Criterion 5

The Consequences of Breakdown in Relationships on Health and Well-Being

Looking back at the first element, we examined physical, intellectual, emotional and social development. Now we will see how these four are affected when relationships break down, in other words, how our health and well-being might suffer.

The table on p.106 outlines the possible affects of relationships breaking down, considering various aspects of peoples lives. Responses vary in strength and duration depending on the individuals concerned and their stages of development, and the importance of the relationship to them.

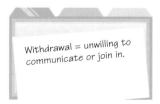

Withdrawal = unwilling to communicate or join in.

Small children and people who cannot express themselves are especially likely to show their responses through their behaviour. It is important for carers to understand this, as changed habits may be explained by some underlying stress related to a breakdown in relationships.

The four lists in the table suggest that the effects of relationship changes are all bad. However, relationships can change for the good, in which case all four areas are still affected, but in a positive way.

1. Effects on emotional life	2. Effects on social life
Withdrawal	Not getting out of bed
Outburst of temper	Staying at home from work or school
Unable to relate to people	Not coming home at night
Loss of trust	Not wanting to go out
Low self-esteem	Change of habits
	Change in language and speech

3. Effects on intellectual activity	4. Effects on physical habits
Loss of motivation	Change in eating habits
Becoming workaholic (working too hard)	Altered sleep patterns
Regression (children going back a stage)	Hyperactivity
Low attention span (cannot concentrate for long)	Weight loss or gain
Stress	Eating disorders (anorexia, bulimia)
Mental illness	Regression (thumb sucking, bedwetting)
Depression	Rocking or head banging
	Violence
	Drug or alcohol abuse

Possible effects of relationships breaking down

ACTIVITY 7

1 Think about two changes in relationships you have experienced, one which you felt bad about, one which you felt good about.

2 Make a list of the effects each of them had on you.

3 Sort them into four categories – emotional, social, intellectual and physical. You will find that the effects overlap and relate to one another in complex ways.

The financial effects of divorce, and homelessness as a result of leaving home, are two examples of the far-reaching changes which altered relationships bring about.

Divorce

- The number of divorces has doubled since 1971, and almost 25% of children are affected by divorce by the age of 16. Divorce of couples with young children is common, and the number of children below 5 affected in 1992 was 57,000, two thirds higher than 1977.

- The proportion of families headed by a lone parent increased from 8% in 1971 to 21% in 1992, although it is important to realise that government statistics do not differentiate between single parents who have never married and parents who have been divorced.

- In 1992, 1 in 5 mothers with dependent children were the sole parent. The percentage of lone fathers was under 2% of all families with dependent children.

- Lone parents comprise 15% of the households in the lowest earning groups, and 1% in the highest earning social group.

- State benefits are targeted on the lower earning groups.

- Benefit expenditure on families with a lone parent rose from 2.6 billion pounds in 1970 to 12.2 billion pounds in 1990. (£ billion at 1993/4 prices)

Leaving home

- In 1993 40,000 households applied to be accepted as homeless. Half were found to have priority needs and housing was provided.

- The percentage of people classed as having parents, relatives or friends no longer able or willing to accommodate them rose from 16% in 1981 to more than 20% in 1993.

- Until they are 18, it is difficult for young people to claim from social security.

- Many young homeless people have been in the care of social services and have no parental home.

- Some young people who leave home do so to avoid physical, emotional or sexual abuse by the family.

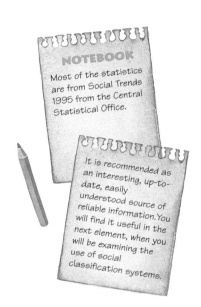

NOTEBOOK

Most of the statistics are from Social Trends 1995 from the Central Statistical Office.

It is recommended as an interesting, up-to-date, easily understood source of reliable information. You will find it useful in the next element, when you will be examining the use of social classification systems.

unit two

ACTIVITY 8

From the information given here, what conclusions might be drawn about

a the financial effects of divorce on families

b the likelihood of homelessness among teenagers who leave home.

Case Studies

You will be continuing to develop the case studies begun in Element 2.1.

Case study 1   The Thatched Cottage

As a child, Rosa was isolated by her deafness. Her twin sister has remained a source of strength all her life. To them both, their religious faith has been a focal point for their friendships; their father was a vicar Rosa's husband enjoys listening to music, but Rosa, of course, cannot share his pleasure; she used to enjoy reading and writing poetry before she became too confused.

Case study 2   Netherfield Community Care

Mishka has developed a friendship with the eccentric caretaker of her block of flats. Debbie cannot understand why they get on – Mishka is proudly Polish, the man is English. Mishka is rather aristocratic and reserved, the caretaker is, quite frankly, rather scruffy and outward going. He accepts Mishka's son's illness calmly, and lets him sleep in the boiler-room when the weather is poor.

Case study 3   Down Way School

Jalwinder and Tim are getting to know one another well. She helps him to cut up his lunch and ties his shoe laces. When there is a dispute in the playground, he runs to her for support, as he is frightened of being bullied. Isabel recommends to Jalwinder that she should encourage Tim to be more independent. He has an imaginary friend who lives at the bottom of the garden and never comes into the house until it is dark. His mother has been asking Isabel if she 'ought to do something' about the friend, as Tim talks to 'it' at night and it is getting on her nerves.

Task 1

1 Work out the most significant relationships for each of the three clients at present.

2 From what you have learnt about them in the case studies, describe what might have happened in the lives of Rosa, Mishka and Tim recently to effect their established relationships.

Task 1

3 How might Rosa's family have been important during her development, both in childhood and after her marriage? As far as you can tell from what you know about them, how might this compare with the impact of the family on Mishka and Tim?

Task 1

4 What might Mishka's reasons be for striking up a friendship with the caretaker? Work out whether they are emotional, intellectual, social, or a combination.

Task 1

5 If Jalwinder stands back from Tim as Isabel suggests, and his mother spirits away his imaginary friend, what might the consequences be for Tim in terms of a breakdown in relationships?

Extension opportunity

When clients first become known to the caring services, it is common for very little to be known about the relationships which are important to them, in either a negative or a positive way.

Task 2

Describe some of the ways in which carers could learn quickly about the most significant relationships of those for whom they become responsible. Explore what might be the negative and positive aspects of the relationships.

Task 2

How might this improve the client/carer relationship?

Discuss these issues and word process your findings, save on a disk and print. [IT 2.1, 2.2]

Multiple Choice Questions

1 Which of the following pairs describes a **formal** relationship?

   a friend/enemy

   b mother/father

   c employer/employee

   d peer/student

2 Which of the following phrases **best** describes the contexts within which relationships are formed

   a the effect of separation from friends

   b the emotions we feel within our family

   c the main areas within which we interact with others

   d the ways in which we manage change

3 The role of the family is to support, provide and

   a promote

   b protect

   c produce

   d procure

4 An eating disorder may be the result of

   a a breakdown in relationships

   b a low fat diet

   c loss of weight

   d emotional security

5 The relationship between a child and parent changes at adolescence because of

   a the parent and child communicating

   b the child understanding the parent

   c parents not understanding each other

   d the child becoming more independent

6 The stress of a relationship breaking down can show itself by changes in

   a predictable events

   b sleeping patterns

   c employment

   d informal groups.

7 Employers and employees have a relationship in

   a a social context

   b a work context

   c a family context

   d an informal context

8 When an employee is promoted, this may cause a change in

   a the context of the voluntary group

   b the consequences of a breakdown in relationships

   c the informal relationship between colleagues

   d the predictable events which affect people's lives

Summary of Evidence Opportunities and Their Relationship to Performance Criteria

Activities 1, 2 and 3	pc 1	**Activity 7**	pc 5
Activity 4	pc 2	**Case studies**	pcs 2, 3, 4 and 5
Activities 5 and 6	pc 3		

Unit 2 element 2 Summary of Element Range and Personal Evidence Tracking Record

Element range references *(tick against left-hand column)*	Description of evidence	Pc and range covered	Portfolio reference number
Pc 1 Relationships			
family – between parents			
– between parents and children			
– between children			
– with the wider family			
at work – formal			
– informal			
social – formal			
–informal			
Contexts of daily life			
family			
work			
social			
Pc 2 Causes of change			
stages in life – infancy to childhood			
– adolescence			
– adulthood			
– midlife			
– old age			
major events – predictable			
– unpredictable			
Pc 3 Reasons for forming relationships			
emotional			
intellectual			
social			
Pc 4			
Role of the family			
protecting			
providing			
supporting			

unit two

Unit 2 element 2 Summary of Element Range and Personal Evidence Tracking Record

Element range references (tick against left-hand column)	Description of evidence	Pc and range covered	Portfolio reference number
Pc 5 Consequences of breakdown in relationships			
effects on – emotional life			
– social life			
– intellectual activity			
– physical habits			

Element 2.3

Explore the Interaction of Individuals within Society and How they may Influence Health and Well-Being

Performance Criteria		
pc 1	Identify the different roles which individuals take within different group settings	113
pc 2	Describe how laws, rules and social conventions affect the roles of individuals	117
pc 3	Compare the characteristics of different social and economic groups using a standard classification system	119
pc 4	Identify the possible impact of the characteristics on individual choices which affect health and well-being	124
pc 5	Assess the classification used	124
	Summary of evidence opportunities and their relationship to the pcs	127
	Summary of element range and personal evidence tracking record	127

unit two

Introduction

In this element we look at the ways in which individuals interact within society, and the different roles played by people within their families, with their friends, and in society as a whole. We examine the ways in which laws, rules and conventions affect those roles.

Individuals are able to make choices within society, and their way of life, health and well-being is affected by those choices. Many social circumstances determine which choices might be made. These circumstances are analysed using standard classification systems.

Finally, ways of scrutinising and analysing the standard classification systems themselves are suggested, so that you can develop the ability to estimate the value of data and information supplied by others.

Performance Criterion 1

The Different Roles which Individuals Take within Different Group Settings

In our interaction within our many and varied relationships, we perceive ourselves to have a **role**. This means a function, or a part that we play as if we were on stage. Sometimes within a single day we take on several different roles as we move from group to group.

When a new member joins a group, his or her role may not be immediately clear, so for a while relationships within the group may be strained until roles are established and members become familiar with the new group structure.

Roles occur within the family, at work, in recreation, and in the community.

Different roles with different groups

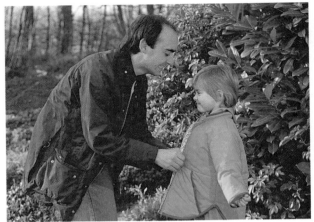

family (father)

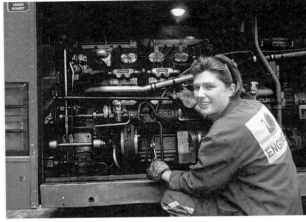

work (mechanic)

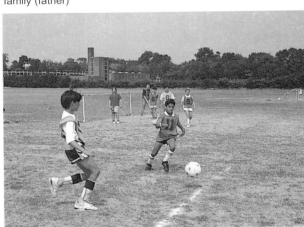

recreation (footballer)

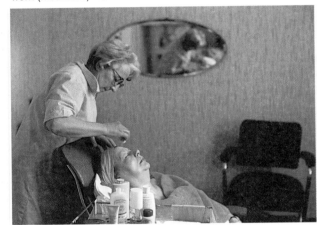

community (neighbour – hairdressing)

How these people behave depends on their views of the role which goes with that label. Their view will have been moulded by the views of those around them, especially those of their families.

Roles in the family

In Activity 1 of Element 2.2 (page 98), you worked out the relationships of members of your family. The woman who has the role of your mother also has the role of wife or partner. If your maternal grandmother is still alive, your mother will also have the role of a daughter, the child of your grandmother. And she will also be your cousin's aunt.

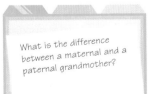

What is the difference between a maternal and a paternal grandmother?

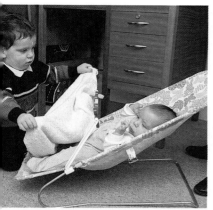

The little mother

Family roles are further complicated by the behaviour tolerated or expected by other members; children are allowed to be childish, mothers are expected to be maternal and caring. Thus if one of the children fulfils a caring role in the family, he or she may be said to be acting like a mother.

If grandparents become dependent on their families, say, for example, after suffering a stroke, roles are reversed and their children may end up having to act like parents, washing, feeding, and changing them as if they were their own children. Such shifting and interchange of roles causes much upheaval in family relationships, as it may take those concerned some time to become adjusted.

Within the family, there is, of course, also room for the role of friend or opponent. There are people whom we meet who impress us, either favourably or unfavourably.

'I want to grow up to be just like him.'

'I will never behave like that.'

Sometimes we do not know where these ideas come from, or we may consciously set out to be like or unlike a specific person. Such people are our **role models**.

Our earliest impressions are of the family, so it is likely that the strongest role models come from within the family structure. This is why family patterns of behaviour emerge. The behaviour is learnt from the role model. Typical family patterns of behaviour include:

- marrying at a certain age
- wearing certain clothes
- laughing in a certain way and at certain things
- eating certain foods
- spending money in a certain fashion.

As we grow independent of our family we take role models from a wider area – pop stars, teachers, friends, work colleagues. Often we choose our role in an attempt to meet the expectations of other people, family, or teachers. Thus our ideas and habits gradually expand. Behaviour patterns learnt when we are very young are powerful, and often stay with us into old age. This puts an enormous responsibility on parents.

When extended families remain close to each other, members often help out with the upbringing of children. Such children have the opportunity to copy a range of personalities from these relationships. This is still the case in many cultures.

Where families are fragmented and scattered, responsibility for rearing children rests with a smaller number of people – maybe only one – who have to take sole responsibility for setting a role model. Children may then look outside the family and identify with teachers or friends as well as the parent or parents.

unit two

ACTIVITY 1

Work out and record in a suitable way the family roles of **a** yourself, **b** your father, and **c** an uncle or aunt.

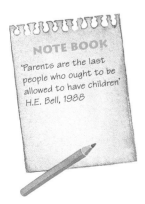

NOTE BOOK

'Parents are the last people who ought to be allowed to have children'
H.E. Bell, 1988

ACTIVITY 2

1 Imagine what would happen if you changed places with
   a your teacher/lecturer
   b one of your parents
   c your local shopkeeper.

2 Discuss how you think your interpretation of their role would compare with their own interpretation.

Roles at work

In the last element we looked at relationships at work, that of employer and employee, and the range of formality/informality between the two. We talk about '**job roles**'; an employee cannot work effectively if it is not clear what is meant to be carried out, what that person's job role is.

Employers will have their idea of what role is to be fulfilled. If it is not shared with the employee then there is confusion, unhappiness and satisfactory relationships cannot be established.

If an employee is promoted, there is a shift of relationships with former colleagues and the employer, and everything is unsettled until new roles and relationships are established. This is more complex when a former employee becomes the employer, and everybody's understanding of roles is turned upside down.

Some people behave as stereotypes of their job, and lose their personal identity when they are at work.

What shall I be today?

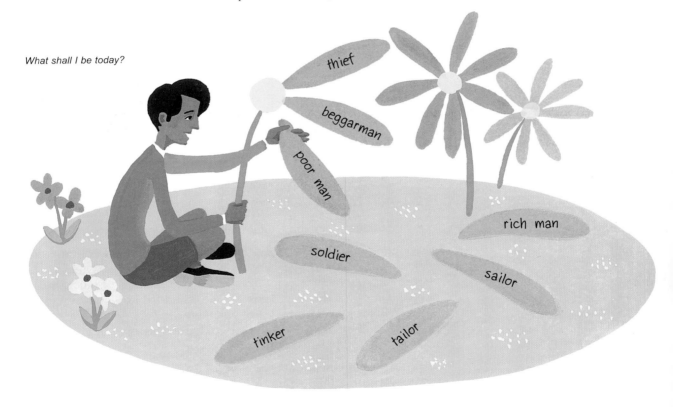

Roles in recreation

Recreation is defined as amusement or relaxation. It includes many different activities, some carried out alone, such as sewing, gardening, watching television, and others in groups, such as team games, going to the pub, dancing. It is the group activities which create the clearest roles:

ACTIVITY 3

1 Can you add any other recreational roles to this list?

2 What roles can you think of which apply to you and any recreational groups you belong to? (Remember that groups may be either formally or informally structured.)

3 Devise a survey from a wide cross-section of individuals to establish their main recreational roles in life.

4 Present your results in an appropriate form to illustrate your conclusions. [NUM 2.1, 2.3]

leader	joker	mate
organiser	confidant	critic
team member	onlooker	peacemaker
partner	best friend	trouble-maker

Roles in the community

Society is the community as a whole, and we are all members of our immediate and wider community. Within it we travel on public transport, go to the shops, use the roads, and so on. Our relationship with others in the community may be more distant than those forged at home, at work, or during our spare time, or they may be quite close, if work in the community becomes an important part of our life.

Some people take up important positions in the community, either out of a sense of responsibility, duty or concern, or as a means of gaining power (which is not always a negative motive). At some stage in our lives we all could be neighbours, tax payers, voters, and service users. By choice we could become community leaders, members of action groups, magistrates, and voluntary workers. Can you think of any other community roles?

unit two

Performance Criterion 2

How Laws, Rules and Social Conventions Affect the Roles of Individuals

Having identified four contexts within which individuals can take different roles, we move on to see what affects the shape of these roles. Laws, rules, and conventions are the three socially based influences we will look at.

Laws

In the United Kingdom, Parliament decides what is to become law, and has to approve any alterations to existing laws. The police and local magistrates' courts enforce the law at a local level. Breaking the law is discouraged by **penalties** such as fines or imprisonment.

Rules

Every culture has accepted rules of behaviour. They set standards and keep communities stable, and are not usually written down. Most people conform to the rules of the society in which they live. If they break the rules of their community, they may be **ostracised**.

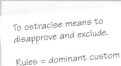

To ostracise means to disapprove and exclude.

Rules = dominant custom

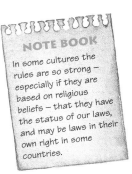

NOTE BOOK

In some cultures the rules are so strong – especially if they are based on religious beliefs – that they have the status of our laws, and may be laws in their own right in some countries.

The effect of rule on roles

The rules of communities are deep and fundamental. Sometimes they are unwritten and unspoken. Sometimes, especially in religious communities, rules are formalised. These often mould cultural habits and rituals, for example arranged marriages, not eating certain foods, wearing particular types of clothing, and attitudes to other members of the family.

If unwritten **rules** are so important that forgetting or ignoring them begins to make life difficult for others, they may be formalised to become **laws**.

Examples of conventions, rules and laws in different contexts

Family

Examples of family **conventions**:

- eating meals at the table, or in front of the television
- what time people are expected to get out of bed
- attitudes to parents and siblings
- whether quarrelling is acceptable
- frequency of family gatherings.

Examples of family **rules**:

- being home by 11pm
- being prompt for meals
- attendance at a place of worship
- no loud music after 10pm
- everybody helps with the chores.

the **laws** specifically related to the family are those of incest.

Work

Examples of work **conventions**:

- use of space
- how people are addressed
- which chair people sit in
- the mugs they drink out of

Examples of work **rules**:

- whether smoking is allowed
- code of dress
- punctuality

Examples of **laws** applying to the workplace:

- safety regulations – HASAW = Health and Safety at work
- laws concerning sex discrimination
- equal opportunities
- who is allowed to do certain tasks
- age-related activities.

Recreation

Examples of **conventions** regarding recreation mainly concern:

- age – 'old ladies don't hang-glide'
- gender – 'boys don't go to needlework classes'
- ability – 'people in wheelchairs don't run races'

Examples of **rules** applying to recreations:

- those peculiar to each game or sport
- fairness and safety rules
- naturally imposed rules – eg plants need watering.

Laws concerned with recreation are similar to those applying at work.

Society

Examples of **conventions** of some societies:

- the celebration of anniversaries, weddings etc
- sending cards at Christmas
- taking a summer break

Note – these are rapidly changing as old patterns of society are being challenged, such as Sunday shopping being permissible and sport spreading from Saturday throughout the week.

Examples of **rules** of some societies:

- buses stop at bus stops
- noise levels should not be too loud at night
- urinating in the street is not acceptable.

*Note – some of these rules have given rise to **by-laws**, that is, laws particular to a district.*

All **laws** apply to the societies within each country.

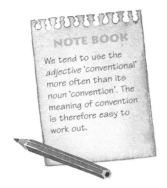

Conventions

Society expects people to behave in certain established ways. In the last few decades many of our traditions and conventions have been challenged as it becomes more acceptable for people to behave as individuals instead of conforming to stereotyped expectations.

This is not the case throughout the world, as societies and cultures change at different rates according to their history and traditions. In rural communities things may not have changed for hundreds of years. Within the United Kingdom the change takes place at varying speeds depending on communications, amount of contact with the outside world, and each community's desire or need for change. When conventions are broken, society shows **disapproval**.

NOTE BOOK

We tend to use the adjective 'conventional' more often than its noun 'convention'. The meaning of convention is therefore easy to work out.

ACTIVITY 4

Select one role from each of the four categories – that is, family, work, recreation, community. Use your work from previous activities in this element and add to them if you need to.

How might each of the roles you have chosen be affected by conventions of dress, culture, age and gender.

◀▶ **Extension opportunity**

Express any opinions in your written account by the use of percentages and average indicators where relevant. [NUM 2.2]

NOTE BOOK

Conventions, rules and laws constrain people's hopes and aspirations, thus affecting the roles they play in life, and whether or not they can be fulfilled easily or only after a struggle.

A **convention** is something which is done with the approval of the majority of people in a community. If it is done often enough, it may become a **rule**. The table opposite lists some examples of conventions, rules and laws in different contexts.

Performance Criterion 3

Comparing Characteristics of Different Social and Economic Groups using a Standard Classification System

Social class classification

In order to make comparisons between social and economic groups objectively, several classification systems are in existence. Traditionally the main access to opportunities is through occupation, and this has become the principal way of dividing people into social classes.

With high unemployment in society today, class divisions are more complex. For your work here, however, this needs to be put aside so that you can choose from the classifications which have been devised and are available for reference. You will be looking at their strengths and weaknesses in pc 5.

Each classification system has a code.

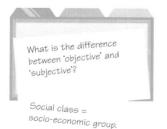

What is the difference between 'objective' and 'subjective'?

Social class = socio-economic group.

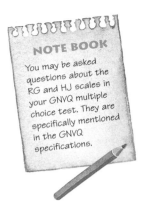

Code	Source
DE	Dept. of Employment
FES	Family Expenditure Survey
HJ	Hall-Jones
HG	Hope-Goldthorpe
MR	Market Research
NS	National Survey
RG	Registrar General's Social Class
RGSEG	Registrar General's Socio-economic Group

Codes used for social class classifications

You need to select *one* of the classifications in order to make the comparisons required by this performance criteria. For example three social classification systems are shown in the table below. You must use *only one* to decide what you mean when you talk about social classes. It's a bit like cooking – you need to use a standard measure or weight throughout the recipe, not mixing ounces with grams, which would make the result a disaster. They are modified from time to time, so make sure you know the date of the system you choose.

Three social classification systems

1 Registrar-General's Scale

I	Professional occupations
II	Intermediate occupations (including most managerial and senior administrative occupations)
IIIN (or a)	Skilled occupations (non-manual)
IIIM (or b)	Skilled occupations (manual)
IV	Partly skilled occupations
V	Unskilled occupations (the armed forces, students, and those whose occupation is inadequately described are listed separately)

2 Hall-Jones Scale

Social Class 1 and 2	The same as the Registrar General's Scale I and II
Social Class 3	Inspectional, supervisory and other non-manual, higher grade
Social Class 4	Inspectional, supervisory and other non-manual, lower grade
Social Class 5	Skilled manual and routine grades of non-manual
Social Class 6	As Registrar General's IV
Social Class 7	As Registrar General's V

3 Market Research

A   Upper middle class – successful business persons (e.g. self-employed/manager/executive of large enterprise); higher professionals (e.g. bishop, surgeon/specialist, barrister, accountant); senior civil servants (above principal) and local government officers (e.g. chief, treasurer, town clerk)

B   Middle class – senior, but not the very top, people in same areas as A

C1 Lower middle class – small tradespeople, non-manual, routine administrative, supervisory and clerical (sometimes referred to as 'white collar' workers)

C2 Skilled working class

D   Semi-skilled and unskilled working class

E   Those at the lowest levels of subsistence including OAPs, those on social security because of sickness or unemployment, and casual workers

The most commonly used in sociology are the Registrar General's (RG) and the Hall-Jones (HJ) systems. In ordinary conversations people are more likely to use the language of the Market Research Scales (MR). The table below compares the RG, HJ and MR scales.

Approximate comparison of social/economic groups according to 3 classifications

Registrar General's	Hall-Jones scale	MR scale
In the UK, this class is too small to be considered on a recognised scale.		Upper class
1	1	A Upper middle class
II	2	B Middle class
IIIN (or a)	3	C1 Lower middle class - 'white collar workers'
	4	
IIIM (or b)	5	C2 Skilled working class
IV	6	D Semi-skilled and unskilled working class
V	7	
Armed forces, students and some others listed separately		E Those at the lowest level of subsistence

unit two

ACTIVITY 5

Use the table at the end of the activity on p.122 to help with this activity.

1 Select *one* of the classification systems after making sure that you have access to information about it.

2 Make a list of the social and economic (class) groups it defines.

3 Compare the following five characteristics of each group:

   • housing

   • environment

   • education

   • employment

   • financial status.

4 Make a note of any aspects of this activity which are confusing or difficult – you will need it in pc 5 – for instance, you may find that the system used contradicts your own experience or opinions.

5 Conduct a survey among a small group of people. Classify them into socio-economic groups using the criteria employed by the classification system you have selected.

6 Illustrate the results in a pictorial form. **[IT 2.1, 2.2, 2.3; NUM 2.1, 2.3]**

7 Break down the survey into the five characteristics listed in step 3. Compare each socio-economic group in a graphical way wherever possible. **[NUM 2.1, 2.3]**

Aspects of the five characteristics

1 Housing

Aspects to consider

- owner-occupied (lived in by the owner who has brought outright or can pay a mortgage)
- rented (from someone on the premises or living away – 'absentee landlord')
- detached
- semi-detached
- terraced
- a house
- a bungalow
- a flat
- a maisonette
- have a garden
- do not have a garden
- travelling people moving from place to place
- no settled address.

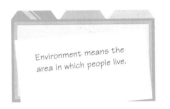

Environment means the area in which people live.

2 Environment

Aspects to consider:

a suburban means on the outskirts of the town

b rural means in the countryside
- high travel costs to work
- homes may be rented or owner-occupied.
- access to shops, community, friends and family.

c urban means in towns
- ability to buy own house
- restrictions of amount of rented accommodation available
- low travel costs to work.
- restriction by local authority residence requirements.

d inner cities mainly concern Birmingham, Liverpool, Manchester, Newcastle and areas of London
- created by massive population increase in the nineteenth century
- density of population remains, properties are old and need renovating
- absentee landlords may not want to spend money on improvements
- shared accommodation in different storeys
- elderly people not wishing to renovate
- access, congestion and crime may discourage the creation of new job opportunities.
- many demands on social and health services

Some inner city areas develop a village-like culture which makes life for its residents more community-oriented and settled.

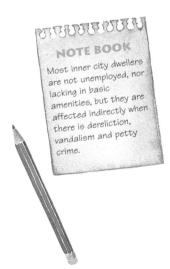

NOTE BOOK

Most inner city dwellers are not unemployed, nor lacking in basic amenities, but they are affected indirectly when there is dereliction, vandalism and petty crime.

3 Education

Aspects to consider:
- encourages the learning of basic skills of reading and numeracy
- passes on social patterns of behaviour from one generation to the next
- prepares people for work
- ethnic groups – language difficulties affect education of children / communication with parents
- situation of schools

- type of school
  public
  private
  state
  boarding or day
  single sex or co-educational
  selective (ie grammar) or comprehensive
  age based – nursery up to the age of 5
    - primary 5–11
    - secondary 11–16 or 18
    - further education (FE) 16–18
    - higher education (HE) 18 upwards
    - adult education
- qualifications currently available
  Post 16 = GCSE, GNVQ, A level and equivalent, graduate
  Higher education = degree or equivalent, or non-graduate qualifications gained at HE institutions.
  Boundaries are blurred as establishments franchise and widen the selection of courses they offer.

4 Employment

Aspects to consider:
- inner city addresses can influence job selection
- distance and cost of transport to work each day
- language
- culture
- ambition
- education
- qualifications
- motivation
- family responsibilities
- other demands on energy, emotions, finances.

5 Financial Status

Aspects to consider
- low income elderly
- low income families
- lowest skilled/least well paid
- low income groups are most prone to ill health
- immigrants may not understand how to gain access to benefits or apply for work
- people earning more money than they need for day-to-day living have disposable income, which means that they have spare money they can spend on holidays, treats, house improvements and investment.
- the opposite is true of low income families

This can lead to
- an upward spiral of increased success for those with a reasonable income and access to opportunity.
- a downward spiral of poverty for those with a low income and few opportunities.

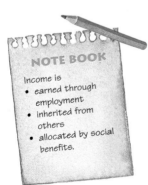

NOTE BOOK

Income is
- earned through employment
- inherited from others
- allocated by social benefits.

Performance Criterion 4

The Possible Impact of the Characteristics on Individual Choices which Affect Health and Well-Being

People's way of life is affected by where they live, how much money they have, whether they have a job or not, and their qualifications. These factors decide how much **choice** there is about lifestyle, health and well-being.

Individual choices

Most people have some degree or choice in the following areas of their lives:

- using health and care services
- nutrition
- alcohol consumption
- smoking habits
- personal hygiene
- exercise

- attitude to education
- maintenance of housing/accommodation
- use of available income – that is, how spending is planned.

ACTIVITY 6

1 Make a chart showing the relationship between the five *characteristics* (housing, environment, education, employment and financial status) and the four *choices* (health, attitude to education, maintenance of housing and use of available income).

2 Use the following scale to indicate the effect of the characteristics on the choices: 1 = low impact, 2 = medium impact, 3 = high impact.

3 Discuss with your colleagues how these choices could affect or have an impact on individuals' health and well-being.

4 Record your conclusions, using ratio/average indicators to emphasise any key findings. **[NUM 2.2]** Use a computer if you wish, or record using images.

Performance Criterion 5

Assessment of the Classification used

In pc 3 (p. 119) you read about standard classification systems and will have used one of them to look at the lifestyles of different socio-economic groups. They all have different strengths and weaknesses. Now you will be working out your opinion of the value and effectiveness of the classification you used.

ACTIVITY 7

1 Discuss in a group how you felt about the classification system you used in terms of:

a **precision**, which means its accuracy

b **omission**, which means anything it missed out

c its **sensitivity to changes in society**

d how much it considers **people's ideas of their own class status**.

2 Record your opinions and those of your colleagues – who may or may not have chosen the same classification system as you.

Case Studies

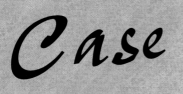

Case study 1   The Thatched Cottage

Mark is analysing Rosa's role in the residential care home. He sees her as a dependent old woman, yet realises that she was once strong and independent. He knows she was lovely too because he has seen photographs of her.

Case study 2   Netherfield Community Care

Debbie finds it hard to work out to which group Mishka may belong. Is it the Polish community, or the residents in the flats, or does she only identify with her son and the caretaker?

Case study 3   Down Way School

Jalwinder has decided that Tim belongs to several groups in which he behaves quite differently. One is that of his classmates, another is that of the adults in his life, and the third is the fantasy world where his friend lives.

Task 1

1   Select two of the clients in one of their roles, or one of the clients in two separate roles.

2   Discuss what these roles are and how they differ from one another.

Task 1

3   What are the factors which affect these roles in terms of conventions, rules and laws?

4   Record your decisions

Multiple Choice Questions

1 Which of the following is a role?

   a class

   b family

   c employee

   d convention

2 Smoking habits, exercise and personal hygiene are examples of

   a health choices

   b education

   c recreation

   d factors

3 The Registrar General's Scale classifies people according to their

   a social class

   b occupation

   c income

   d education

4 Standard classification systems are assessed in terms of their

   a classification, recommendations, revision

   b effectiveness, provision of detail, accuracy

   c precision, omissions, sensitivity to change

   d reputation, sensitivity, reflection of society

5 At different time in life, the same person could be a

   a parent, daughter, husband

   b mother, maternal grandparent, nephew

   c child, father, cousin

   d wife, sibling, paternal grandfather

6 A magistrate holds a role in

   a recreation

   b work

   c the family

   d the community

7 Using a saucer with a cup is an example of

   a a social convention

   b a safety regulation

   c a workplace law

   d a socio-economic rule

8 Attitudes to education, smoking habits and use of available income are all examples of

   a individual choices

   b housing characteristics

   c conventions affecting individuals

   d use of health and care services

Summary of Evidence Opportunities and Their Relationship to Performance Criteria

Activities 1, 2 and 3	pc 1	Activity 6	pc 4
Activity 4	pc 2	Activity 7	pc 5
Activity 5	pc 3	Case studies	pcs 1 and 2

Unit 2 Element 3 Summary of Element Range and Personal Evidence Tracking Record

Element range references (tick against left-hand column)	Description of evidence	Pc and range covered	Portfolio reference number
Pc 1 Roles and group settings			
family – husband, wife, parent, child			
work – employer, employee			
recreation – organiser, participant,			
community – neighbour, tax payer, voter, service user			
Pc 2 Roles as pc 1			
Pc 3 Characteristics			
housing			
environment			
education			
employment			
financial status			
pc 4 Individual choices			
use of health and care service			
nutrition			
alcohol consumption			
smoking habits			
personal hygiene			
exercise			
attitude to education			
maintenance of housing			
use of available income			
Pc 5 Assessment of social classification scale			
precision			
omission			
sensitivity to change in society			

unit two

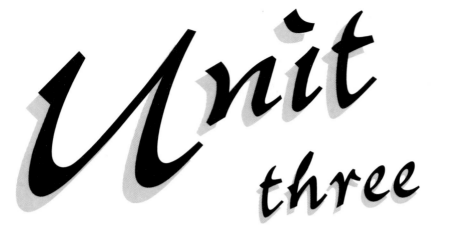

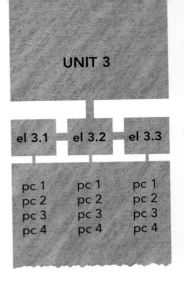

UNIT 3

el 3.1	el 3.2	el 3.3
pc 1	pc 1	pc 1
pc 2	pc 2	pc 2
pc 3	pc 3	pc 3
pc 4	pc 4	pc 4

Health and Social Care Services

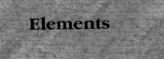

Elements

3.1 Investigate the provision of health and social care services

3.2 Describe how the needs of different clients are met by health and social care services

3.3 Investigate jobs in health and social care

The aim of this unit is to help you to understand the facilities made available through health and social care services.

The first element requires you to look at the services which are available nationally, and how they are reflected in your own area. The second element is about the way in which different client groups can be helped by the care services, how they can get help, and how they become known to the services in the first place. The third element examines the jobs people have in the care services, what they actually do at work, and the qualifications and career paths they have followed.

Element 3.1

Investigate the Provision of Health and Social Care Services

Performance Criteria

pc 1 Explain the organisation of statutory health and social care services   130

pc 2 Describe the health and social care services provided by non-statutory and independent sectors   133

pc 3 Describe the forms of health and social care provided by informal carers   134

pc 4 Explain the methods of funding non-statutory sectors
Improve your local knowledge   135

Summary of evidence opportunities and their relationship to the pcs   143

Summary of element range and personal evidence tracking record   143

Introduction

This element first examines health and social care services provided by the state, and then the services provided in other ways. After finding out who delivers care, you will look at who pays for it, and where the funds come from. The element explains the role of the statutory and non-statutory sectors, and how health and social care services are provided by certain bodies and purchased by others. You will also learn about informal caring by friends, relatives and support groups. The table below summarises the provision of health and social care.

Summary of provision of health and social care

Category	Explanation	Examples
1 Statutory	Provided by the state; that is, services which must be provided by law	NHS Social Services
2 Non-statutory **a** Voluntary	Privately organised, often non-profit making. Filling gaps in state provision	NSPCC, Mind, Help the Aged
b Private	Privately owned and run on business lines – profit-making	BUPA hospitals, private residential care, nursing agencies
c Self-employed	Similar to private, but on smaller scale	Child minders, foster care
d Informal	Provided by the family and community	Family care of disabled child Day services provided by a church group

unit three

A short section explaining regional variations is included, to help you to understand what health and care provision is available in your own area within the national framework.

Performance Criterion 1

The Organisation of Statutory Health and Social Care Services

The National Health Service (NHS) and Local Authority Social Services together form the two branches of the **statutory** services. Both are controlled nationally by the Secretary of State for Health.

The National Health Service

The care given by the NHS may be described as primary care, secondary care, or tertiary care.

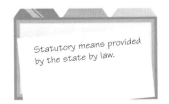

Statutory means provided by the state by law.

The people whom you meet first when you need looking after by the National Health Service offer you **primary care**. Often this is in your GP's surgery or at a health clinic, and includes the GP, the practice nurse and the health visitor.

Sometimes primary care is **preventive**, which may mean that advice is given to stop someone becoming unwell. The promotion of how to stop smoking, and pre-natal care to make sure that a pregnant woman remains in the best possible health until her baby is born are examples. Primary care is always given outside hospitals, in the community.

Secondary care is always given in hospitals. If you went to an Accident and Emergency department of a hospital, you would be going straight into secondary care. If your GP referred you to a hospital consultant, you would be moving from primary into secondary care. Secondary care is usually **curative**, which means it is intended to make you better, or improve your state of health.

The stage following secondary care is called **tertiary care**, tertiary meaning third. It refers to long-term care, which includes rehabilitation.

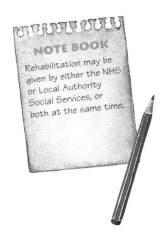

NOTE BOOK

Rehabilitation may be given by either the NHS or Local Authority Social Services, or both at the same time.

Rehabilitation is care intended to restore people to health, or to help them to live as fully as possible within the limits of their personal state of health. This includes, for example,

- those who have had a stroke who may be in tertiary care while they adjust to reduced mobility

- people who have suffered spinal injury who might remain in tertiary care until their condition is stable and they have learnt how to manage ordinary household tasks from a wheelchair.

In 1990, The **NHS and Community Care Act** began the concept of purchasing and providing, with the introduction of independent NHS Trusts, and general practitioner fund holders. This means that some organisations buy in the services they needed from other organisations.

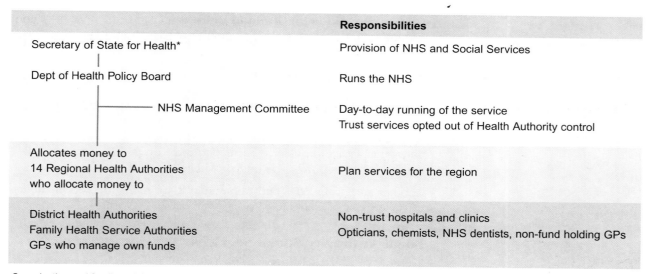

	Responsibilities
Secretary of State for Health*	Provision of NHS and Social Services
Dept of Health Policy Board	Runs the NHS
NHS Management Committee	Day-to-day running of the service Trust services opted out of Health Authority control
Allocates money to 14 Regional Health Authorities who allocate money to	Plan services for the region
District Health Authorities Family Health Service Authorities GPs who manage own funds	Non-trust hospitals and clinics Opticians, chemists, NHS dentists, non-fund holding GPs

Organisation and funding of the NHS in England: three tiers

*There are separate Secretaries of State for Health in Scotland, Wales and Northern Ireland.

Independent NHS Trusts

Trust hospitals can choose to operate their own budgets without consulting health authorities. They are self-governing, while remaining within the NHS. NHS trusts can spend their own money in the ways they think best. They become **providers** of services, such as physiotherapy, which are bought by other **purchasers**, such as fund-holding GPs.

Sometimes NHS Trusts cover a wider field than the hospital alone, maybe joining with clinics and health centres. Thus there are many local variations. You will be looking at those in your own particular area later.

unit three

GPs (purchasers)

1 Fund holders:
- send patient to place which in their opinion, offers the best value
- pays bills up to £5000. Above this, the area Health Authority pays

2 Non-fund holders:
- send patients to places with which the area Health Authority has a contract
- the area Health Authority pays

Hospitals (may be purchasers or providers)

1 Trust hospitals:
- compete to treat patients

2 Non-Trust hospitals:
- are run by Area Health Authorities
- compete for contracts to run health care services
- are paid by Area Health Authorities or fund-holding GPs

3 Private:
- are paid by individuals
- costs may be covered by insurance
- fund-holding GPs or area Health Authorities may pay for services

Purchaser and providers in the NHS

General Practitioner (GP) fund holders

A **general practitioner** is a family doctor. If a GP chooses to become a fund holder, the money allocated by the Regional Health Authority can be spent on hospitals and other services as the doctor chooses.

From the first table on p. 131 you will be able to trace the provision of funds from national down to area level. You will also see where the money given to hospitals and GPs funded in different ways comes from. Remember that in some cases the purchaser can at the same time be a service provider. The second table on p. 131 examines GPs and hospitals as purchasers and providers.

Another aim of the NHS and Community Care Act is to keep members of society out of institutions as far as possible.

Local Authority Social Services

The role of social services is to give advice, give access to services, and provide some services, including community and residential care. Local Authority Social Services departments purchase services from the full range of statutory, and non-statutory providers. (See also pc 2.)

Personal social services make provision for

- families
- children
- young people
- adults
- clients with physical disabilities
- people with learning difficulties and disabilities
- elderly people.

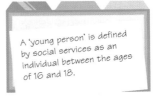

A 'young person' is defined by social services as an individual between the ages of 16 and 18.

The organisers responsible for delivering care have to work together to make sure that standards are high and that money is spent wisely. In order to make sure that providers are chosen effectively, the needs of clients have to be **assessed** carefully.

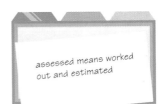

assessed means worked out and estimated

Community services are provided either by Local Authority Social Services or the NHS, or by both working together. Their aim is to deliver care within the community or in the clients' own homes. Workers in the area of community service include:

- community nurses
- social services field workers
- community psychiatric nurses
- midwives.

Finance

Half of all state spending is on health and social care and the government finances statutory health and social care services through central and local government (See the table opposite).

Government sources	
Central government	• from income tax (**'fiscal measures'**) • National insurance contributions (from employers and employees) • charges on dental and optical services and prescriptions
Local government	• from support grants and local taxes

Financing of statutory health and social care services

Performance Criterion 2

The Health and Social Care Services Provided by Non-Statutory and Independent Sectors

You will be looking at the services offered by different agencies covering **voluntary**, **private** and **self-employed** care. These are the **non-statutory** services, which means that they are not provided by the state.

ACTIVITY 1

Write down the main purpose of the six voluntary organisations mentioned on the right.

The voluntary sector

This sector is made up of organisations usually described as charities. They often fill some gap in care which is not totally filled by the statutory services, such as the Women's Royal Voluntary Service, Save the Children Fund, and Barnardos. Others provide funding, support or care connected with specific conditions, such as the Terence Higgins Trust, the Chest, Heart and Stroke Association, and Scope.

The private sector

The private sector is made up of organisations run for a profit, such as private hospitals, for example those run by BUPA, private residential care homes, and private nursery schools and playgroups.

The self-employed sector

Individuals who might be paid **either** by those who choose to pay for care **or** by social services make up the self-employed sector, and includes childminders, and those providing foster care.

unit three

ACTIVITY 2

1 Make three lists of care services providers in your area, under the headings 'voluntary', 'private' and 'self-employed'.

2 Which list is the longest?

3 Can you draw any conclusion from this?

4 Conduct a survey among a wide cross-section of individuals to ascertain what they consider to be the most important service offered in the three categories. Use graphical illustrations and probability terms to support the conclusions. **[NUM 2.1, 2.3]**

5 How does the result of your survey compare with local provision as listed in step 2?

6 Discuss the comparison in your group.

Performance Criterion 3

Forms of Health and Social Care Provided by Informal Carers

An **informal carer** is one who receives no formal payment for services in the form of nursing, companionship, and help in the home. Examples of each of these are

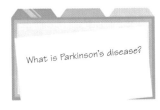

What is Parkinson's disease?

- a husband caring for his wife who suffers from Parkinson's disease
- a neighbour dropping in for coffee and a chat with a housebound friend
- children shopping for invalid parents.

From these examples it will be easy for you to work out that informal carers include children, parents, friends and neighbours, and local support groups.

Children are a growing group of carers as it becomes more common for people with disabilities to have families. Some of the children begin in their caring role at a very early age. They may also be expected to help if there is a sibling who needs care in the family. Adult children often look after elderly parents.

Parents are frequently the main carers if a child (or children) need constant attention.

Friends and neighbours often rally round to help someone who lives alone and is in need of support.

Local support groups can be a source of help to families and individuals, and may be part of a religious or cultural group, or part of a national charity.

Informal carers are entitled to, and are usually deserving of, all the help available from their local community services. This is why you will be examining how clients and client groups can be referred to health and social care services in Element 3.2.

If you choose to go into health and social care work, you may find that members of the public ask you for advice. When you have studied Element 3.2 you will understand how informal carers can gain access to help and support from statutory and non-statutory services, and be able to give information which is accurate and helpful

ACTIVITY 3

1 Working as a group, discuss any examples of informal caring which you know about.

2 Make a diagram showing
  a the form of care provided
  b by whom it is provided.

Performance Criterion 4

The Methods of Funding Non-Statutory Sectors

Within the provision described in the first three performance criteria, we now need to see how costs can be covered for individuals or groups seeking access to services provided by the non-statutory sectors.

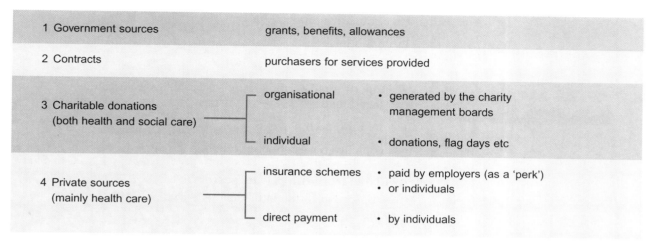

| 1 Government sources | grants, benefits, allowances |
| 2 Contracts | purchasers for services provided |

3 Charitable donations (both health and social care)
- organisational — • generated by the charity management boards
- individual — • donations, flag days etc

4 Private sources (mainly health care)
- insurance schemes — • paid by employers (as a 'perk') • or individuals
- direct payment — • by individuals

Summary

To draw this rather complex element to a close, here is a summary of health and social care services in the United Kingdom:

Examples of services available from the various sectors providing health and social care

1 Available from the NHS

a free:

- access to a family doctor (GP)
- casualty department treatment (accident and emergency services)
- acute hospital care (hospital care that is not long term)

b for which a basic fee is paid:

- dentist
- optician
- prescriptions.

Note: fees can be waived through the benefit systems.

2 Available from local authorities

a free:

- services to children and families
- services to those with mental illness – **shared with the NHS**
- probation service

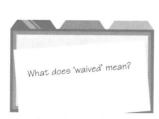

What does 'waived' mean?

b at a cost depending on income:

- day care facilities
- home help services.

3 Available from voluntary organisations

(free, by donation)

Examples include:

- Help the Aged day care
- support from specific groups – Alcoholics Anonymous, Gingerbread
- advice from helplines

Funds come from subscriptions, nationwide appeals, or bequests.

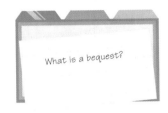

What is a bequest?

4 Available from the private sector

(that is, for which the individual pays, which may or may not be covered by insurance)

- dentist
- osteopath
- private hospital care
- agency services for home care
- residential care.

5 Available from self-employed providers

(paid for either by local authority social services or individuals)

- child minding
- foster care.

6 Provided by the community or family (informal care)

(usually free)

- caring for members of the family
- local support groups – religious, or those filling specific care needs
- friends and neighbours.

So we have seen which services have to be paid for by the individual and which are provided by the state.

Local provision

Having studied the broad outline of national provision, you now need to look at your local scene to understand the health and care provision in your own area.

You will have to gain your knowledge of this by experience, as every student's findings will be different according to where he or she lives. The following activities will guide you through the process, and at the same time provide you with assessable evidence.

National Health Service

Within their national structures, all four countries – England, Northern Ireland, Scotland, Wales – deliver very similar services to their communities.

England   **Secretary of State for Health**
                            Regional Health Authorities
                            District Health Authorities

There are 8 Regional Health Authorities in England, and 3 separate authorities for Wales, Scotland and Ireland (p. 138).

Scotland   **Secretary of State for Scotland**
                            Scottish Home and Health Dept
                            Local Health Boards

The Secretary of State for Scotland is answerable to Parliament for Scottish health services which are administered by the Scottish Home and Health Department. Local Health Boards are responsible for providing services at district level.

Wales   **Secretary of State for Wales**
                            Department of Health
                            District Health Authorities

Organisation of the NHS in Wales is similar to that of England but omitting the Regional Health Authorities.

Northern Ireland   **Department of Health**
                            Local Health Boards

Health services are organised as a single agency outside political control. The Department of Health allocates funding directly to the four local Health Boards.

Organisation of the four National Health Services

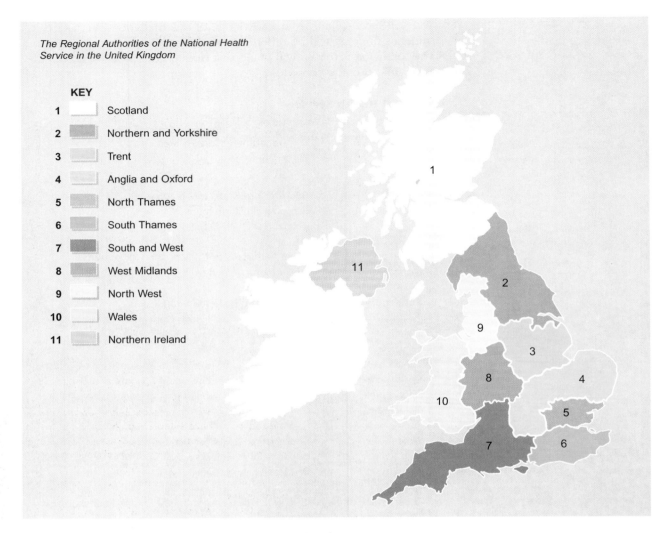

The Regional Authorities of the National Health Service in the United Kingdom

KEY

1	Scotland
2	Northern and Yorkshire
3	Trent
4	Anglia and Oxford
5	North Thames
6	South Thames
7	South and West
8	West Midlands
9	North West
10	Wales
11	Northern Ireland

Social Services

The table below outlines the organisation of social services in the UK.

Organisation of Social Services

	Responsibilities
Secretary of State for Health	Provision of Social Services
Local Authorities*	Administration and co-ordination of social services
Social Services Committee	Social services within its area
* Local Authorities run by: England and Wales – County Councils – Metropolitan district councils – London boroughs	
Northern Ireland – 4 Boards (outside political control)	Administer social and health services
Scotland – Regional Local Authorities	Control social work departments

ACTIVITY 3

◀▶ **Extension opportunity**

Improve your local knowledge

1 Find out the structure of the NHS in your area.

2 Make a diagram similar to p.131 (top), but with names of the departments in your area.

   Compose the diagram using a computer. Save on disk and print. [**IT 2.1, 2.2, 2.3**]

3 Support this with notes containing telephone number and addresses.

4 Who manages the health services in your local area?

5 Are there any local Trusts in you area?

6 Which of the doctors hold their own budgets?

7 Is your own GP a budget holder or not?

8 Can you name any NHS dentists?

Present your findings, incorporating numerical information such as percentages, ratios, fractions or decimal fractions, to support any conclusions and opinions formed. [**NUM 2.2**]

You may choose to use a computer to present the information. [**IT 2.1 2.2 2.3**]

ACTIVITY 4

◀▶ **Extension opportunity**

1 Find out the local structure of Social Services.

2 Make a table like that in the table on page 138, but with actual names of the departments in your area.

   Compose the diagram using a computer. Save on disk and print. [**IT 2.1, 2.2, 2.3**]

3 You will find long lists of local services providers in the Yellow Pages. Make lists under the headings

   • statutory   • self-employed

   • non-statutory   • support for home carers.

   • voluntary

   • private

   Expand the lists you made in Activity 2

4 Draw up some relevant questions which would enable you to compare another county's health and social care with your own. Decide first how you would find answers to your questions. Is there somewhere you can go for help? Do you have access to written information. Conduct research based on the questions you have established. When making comparisons you can present graphical illustrations, compare probabilities and express information in the form of percentages, ratio, and average indicators to support any conclusions which are made about the two counties. [**NUM 2.1, 2.2, 2.3**]

unit three

139

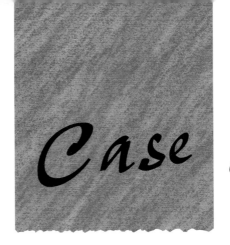

Case Studies

Case study 1   Netherfield Community Care

Mikhail is working with the family of Horace, a frail elderly man, to make sure that he remains supported in his wish to stay independent and living alone. He has asked Debbie to make a diagram for him to use when explaining to Horace's relatives the differences between the statutory, voluntary, self-employed and private sectors which could contribute to Horace's care.

Task 1

Produce the sort of diagram which would be helpful for this purpose.

Case study 2   Hill Hall

The school is run by the Local Authority. Ann is surprised at the variety of services used by the pupils and provided by different organisations.

Task 2

Imagine Hill Hall is in your area.

1   When requiring the following services, which local organisations would be able to provide them?

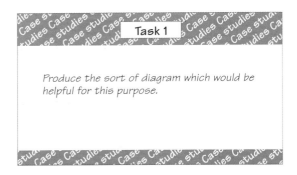

- speech therapy
- catering
- hydrotherapy
- repairs to computers
- supply of continence aids for the clients who are incontinent
- transport to and from home or on outings.

Incontinent means unable to control the passing of urine and/or faeces.

Task 2

2   Who would be the purchaser, who would be the provider, and how would the services be paid for?

Case study 3   The Thatched Cottage

Mark comes back from holiday, and is surprised to see several clients he doesn't recognise in the sitting room. Dora explains that the management is trying out some new systems in order to help the local community. Midday meals are available to those living nearby, some day care facilities are being offered, and when accommodation allows, there will be respite care offered. Local home carers are enthusiastic.

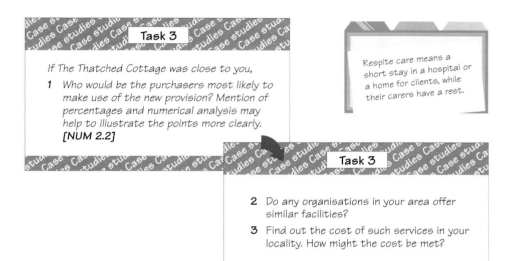

Task 3

If The Thatched Cottage was close to you,

1   Who would be the purchasers most likely to make use of the new provision? Mention of percentages and numerical analysis may help to illustrate the points more clearly. [NUM 2.2]

Respite care means a short stay in a hospital or a home for clients, while their carers have a rest.

Task 3

2   Do any organisations in your area offer similar facilities?
3   Find out the cost of such services in your locality. How might the cost be met?

Case study 4   Down Way School

As part of her course, Jalwinder has to create a booklet which would be of help to new parents. She is keen to make it useful, so she discusses it with Isabel and the class teacher. They suggest that, as there is already a welcome pack for new parents, she should use the opportunity to outline the health and social care facilities available for children in the local community.

Task 4

The welcome pack should be of loose leaflets in a folder with a pocket. Working as a group, design the leaflets Jalwinder could produce if she lived in your locality. The leaflets should have words and pictures, all in the same 'house style', covering each of the following aspects:

- playgroups
- creches
- health clinics
- holiday child care
- local GPs
- places of worship
- libraries
- mother and toddler groups
- any other matters you consider to be important.

Task 4

Print all the leaflets and save on a disk. [IT 2.1, 2.2, 2.3]

Include a map to show where the main places are, including the Citizens' Advice Bureau, Social Services and the nearest post office.

unit three case studies

Multiple Choice Questions

1 The National Health Services mainly provide

    a *recreational care*

    b *health care*

    c *family care*

    d *community care*

2 The services provided by charitable organisations are described as

    a *voluntary*

    b *statutory*

    c *private*

    d *social*

3 Which one of the following statements applying to Trust hospitals is true?

    a *they are under the control of their District Health Authority*

    b *they are answerable to fund-holding GPs*

    c *they are independent of the NHS*

    d *they operate their own budgets*

4 Which of the following is a provider of care?

    a *Local Authorities*

    b *the occupational sector*

    c *Regional authorities*

    d *the insurance sector*

5 When applied to finances, the meaning of 'fiscal' is

    a *money raised from taxation*

    b *charitable donations*

    c *insurance schemes*

    d *payment by individuals*

6 Opticians, NHS dentists, chemists and non-fund holding GPs are all organised by

    a *District Health Authorities*

    b *NHS Authorities*

    c *Area Health Authorities*

    d *Family Health Service Authorities*

7 Informal carers may meet the needs of clients by

    a *providing statutory care*

    b *forming contracts with local providers*

    c *providing primary health care*

    d *forming local support groups*

8 Secondary care may be provided

    a *in hospital wards*

    b *by a practice nurse*

    c *through rehabilitation*

    d *only to elderly people*

Summary of Evidence Opportunities and Their Relationship to Performance Criteria

Activities 1 and 2	pc 2	**Case study 1**	pcs 1 and 2	**Case study 4**	pcs 1, 2 and 3
Activities 3	pc 3	**Case study 2**	pcs 1, 2, 3 and 4		
Activities 4 and 5	pcs 1, 2 and 3	**Case study 3**	pcs 2 and 4		

Unit 3 Element 1 Summary of Element Range and Personal Evidence Tracking Record

Element range reference *(tick against left-hand column)*	Description of evidence	Pc and range covered	Portfolio reference number
Pc 1 Organisation			
overall structure			
– government department level			
– regional level			
– area level			
purchaser and provider			
function of services			
inter-relationship of services			
Statutory health and social care services			
NHS – primary care			
– secondary care			
– tertiary care			
– community services			
personal social services			
– provision for families			
– provision for children			
– provision for young people			
– provision for adults			
– provision for clients with physical disabilities			
– provision for people with learning difficulties and disabilities			
– provision for elderly people			
Pc 2 Non-statutory and independent sectors			
voluntary			
private – hospitals			
– residential homes			
– nursery schools			
self-employed			
– childminders			
– foster carers			

unit three

Unit 3 Element 1 Summary of Element Range and Personal Evidence Tracking Record

Element range references (tick against left-hand column)	Description of evidence	Pc and range covered	Portfolio reference number
Pc 3 Forms of health and social care			
nursing			
companionship			
help in the home			
Informal carers			
children			
parents			
friends			
neighbours			
local support groups			
Pc 4 Methods of funding			
donation			
government grants			
grants			
direct payment			
insurance			

Element 3.2

Describe How the Needs of the Different Clients are Met by Health and Social Care Services

Performance Criteria		
pc 1	Describe the needs of client groups using health and social care services	145
pc 2	Describe the services provided to meet the needs of client groups	149
pc 3	Explain methods of referral to services for different client groups	150
pc 4	Describe support for client groups to make use of services	151
	Summary of evidence opportunities and their relationship to the pcs	157
	Summary of element range and personal evidence tracking record	157

Introduction

Beginning by identifying who requires the services of the community, this element examines the needs of different groups. Next the services which have developed to meet those needs are described, and how people can make contact with them. Lastly the support which will help people to make the best use of the services is explained.

Performance Criterion 1

The Needs of Client Groups Using Health and Social Care Services

The word **client** has developed as a blanket term to describe anybody in need of health and social care. It covers patients in hospital, trainees in sheltered workshops, and all those using health and social care services who have no other neat term to describe them. It is a word with drawbacks, as it is not very warm or friendly, but is an improvement on 'service user' or 'member of the public'.

Client groups

When several clients have similar needs and require similar services, they become members of a **client group**: babies, children, young people, adults, elderly people, and families are examples of client groups. Their **needs** may be

- physical
- mental
- emotional
- social.

unit three

145

Physical needs

Physical needs may be due to disease, physical disability or a learning disability.

Disease

Disease can be either **acute** or **chronic**. Acute means short-term, beginning suddenly with rapid change in the patients condition, or curable; chronic means long-term and persistent with little change from day to day.

ACTIVITY 1

1 In discussion, decide which of the following complaints are **acute**, which are **chronic** and which come into **both categories**. You may need to look up some of the words. *Flu, results of an accident, heart attack, diabetes, epilepsy, measles, stroke, coeliac disease, arthritis, haemophilia, athlete's foot, leprosy, asthma, malaria.*

2 List your decisions under the three headings.

3 Draw up a survey by devising questions which will enable you to ascertain how common the diseases/illnesses are. Present your information in a variety of graphical forms. Express opinions of the graphical displays using probabilities wherever possible. [NUM 2.1, 2.3]

Physical disability

Congenital disability   Our bodies are amazingly complex, and it is no surprise that sometimes during development things go wrong and babies are born with a disability of one degree or another. Such disabilities are said to be **congenital** and can be for **genetic** reasons (inherited) or **environmental** reasons (damage during development in the womb or at birth).

Acquired disabilities   These are disabilities due to illness or injury after birth.

Congenital and acquired disabilities can be either **motor** – to do with movement, or **sensory** – to do with our senses (sight, hearing, touch, taste, smell).

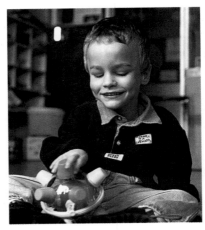

This boy has a congenital disability: he was blind from birth.

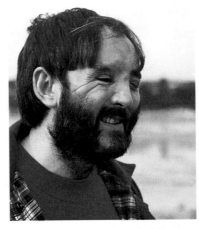

This man has an acquired disability: he lost his sight in an accident.

A syndrome is a group of symptoms.

- learning difficulties
- special needs
- mental disabilities
all mean the same as learning disabilities

ACTIVITY 2

1 In discussion, decide which of the following disabilities are **congenital**, which are **acquired**, and which could be **either**. You may need to look up some of the words.

Cataract, spina bifida, hemiplegia, short-arm syndrome, deafness, cerebral palsy, limb amputation.

2 List your decisions under the three headings.

3 Which are **motor** and which are **sensory** disabilities?

Learning disability

Usually learning disabilities are recognised in childhood, but sometimes they develop as a result of illness or injuries which affect the brain and stop it functioning normally. Learning difficulties are described as being **moderate**, or **severe**, as they range from inability to understand some aspects of daily living to profound dysfunction which could result in death in early adulthood or sooner.

Individuals with learning difficulties may or may not have physical disabilities as well. It is not now considered acceptable to describe people as being mentally handicapped.

Emotional needs

These needs, like physical ones, may be either short or long term, depending on the personality of the client and the nature and extent of the cause. **Trauma** means injury or damage, and it can be either *physical*, as in a cut finger, or *psychological*, as in stress.

When 'dys' is put in front of a word it means that difficulty is involved:

dys-lexia = difficulty with words

dys-pepsia = difficulty with digestion

dys-phagia = difficulty with swallowing

dys-trophy = difficulty with muscle growth.

ACTIVITY 3

Make a list of two possible causes of emotional or psychological trauma which could be experienced by *each* of the six client groups identified earlier: babies, children, young people, adults, elderly people, families.

Examples: Children's emotional needs have to be considered after bereavement; adult groups may be psychologically traumatised after a major incident such as a football stadium tragedy.

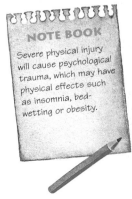

NOTE BOOK

Severe physical injury will cause psychological trauma, which may have physical effects such as insomnia, bed-wetting or obesity.

Mental health needs

Mental health is to the mind what physical health is to the body. You have already seen that psychological and physical trauma are related to each other. In the same way some physical disorders can show themselves with psychological symptoms. Again, mental health disorders can be acute or chronic.

unit three

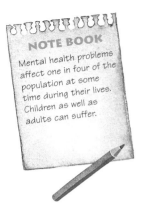

Acute   For example: food allergies can cause behavioural problems in children; hormone imbalance can cause post-natal depression; uncontrolled diabetes can cause aggression. Mental health needs of this nature are treated through the underlying cause. A considerable percentage of mental health illnesses unconnected to physical disorders are short term and curable.

Chronic   For example, schizophrenia, psychotic behaviour, manic depression, obsessions. Many chronic mental health conditions are manageable with medication, although they may not be curable. It can be a problem to make sure that some sufferers take their prescribed drugs, as sometimes their mental state means that they are not able or inclined to do so.

Social needs

All client groups will have social requirements to be met. For example: individuals with physical disabilities may need help with developing self-esteem; families may need support while they adjust to the birth of a baby with disabilities; a child with epilepsy may need guidance through developing friendships. In addition, the main tasks of social service are about supporting families, groups and all individuals

- financially (with benefits)
- emotionally (with personal contact and advice)
- in material ways (with housing, furniture, etc).

Several client groups will have **educational needs** which will have to be addressed at the same time. Examples are children with special needs, and adults with schizophrenia who choose to go to evening classes.

Summary table

Physical	Emotional	Social
• disease	• physical	• financial
• physical disability	• psychological	• emotional
motor/sensory		• material
congenital/acquired	**Mental**	
• learning disability	• acute	
moderate	• chronic	
severe		

Needs of client groups using Health and Social Care Services

Performance Criterion 2

The Services Provided to Meet the Needs of Client Groups

In Element 1, pc 2, you examined the provision of health and social care. Now you are going to see how those services meet the needs of clients. As a reminder the table on the left provides a summary of the headings used in the last element, where provision was discussed.

The figure below lists various client needs and the services available to meet them.

Statutory

1 Services available from the NHS
   a free
   b for which a basic fee is paid (ability to pay is taken into account)

2 Service available from local authorities
   a free
   b at a cost depending on income

Voluntary

Services available from charities

Private

Services for which the individual/family pays

Self-employed

Services for which local authorities or the individual/family pays

Informal

Services provided by the community or family

Client needs and services available

CLIENT NEEDS	NHS	Local Authority	Voluntary	Private	Informal	Self-employed
Physical needs - acute	✓			✓	✓	
- chronic	✓	✓	✓	✓	✓	
Physical disabilities	✓	✓	✓	✓	✓	
Learning disabilities	✓	✓	✓	✓	✓	
Emotional	✓	✓	✓	✓	✓	
Mental health		✓	✓	✓	✓	
Social needs		✓		✓	✓	✓
Benefits		✓			✓	

SERVICES

ACTIVITY 4

Purpose: to work out the relationships between client groups, their needs and services provided.

1 Work out what choices of services are available in your locality to the following client groups:

   a Parents of children with Downs syndrome.

   b Young adults showing signs of schizophrenia.

   c Families whose elderly relatives are becoming increasingly hard of hearing.

   d Young people with fears of HIV.

   e Children contracting meningitis.

   f Adults with cerebral palsy needing residential care.

2 Use a computer to recreate the grid in the figure above. Complete your grid for each client group putting an asterisk (*) where services are available. (You should produce six grids each with the title of a different client group.) **[IT 2.1, 2.2, 2.3]**

You need first to work out which category (physical, emotional, mental or social) their needs come under.

unit three

Performance Criterion 3

Methods of Referral to Services for Different Client Groups

You will examine how services are made available to clients by looking at the four main routes by which they are referred to (put in touch with) services. These are professional referral, self-referral, referral by others, and referral by emergency services, either National Health Services or local services. All of these apply to all services providers –*statutory, voluntary, self-employed* and *private*.

Professional referral

Professional referral involves one professional assessing clients' needs and putting them in touch with another professional or agency. Examples include:

- a GP refers a child with chronic tonsillitis to a hospital ear, nose and throat consultant **(NHS – no fee)**
- a voluntary agency refers a homeless young person to the social services department **(local authority – no fee)**
- a college tutor refers a student with emotional problems to a counselling service **(voluntary or local authority – no fee)**
- a school where a pupil has a record of non-attendance contacts the Education Welfare Officer **(local authority – no fee)**.

Self-referral

Self-referral takes place when someone decides for themselves where to go for help. Examples include:

- a student aged 20 with toothache goes to the dentist **(basic fee – NHS)**
- a mother whose child has chickenpox contacts her GP **(NHS – no fee)**
- an adult with alcohol-related problems attends Alcoholics Anonymous **(voluntary – no fee)**
- a single parent contacts social services to enquire about benefits **(local authority – no fee)**.

Referral by others

Where referral by others is the route this means that another person acts on an individual client's behalf. Examples include:

- neighbours worried about child abuse contact the NSPCC **(voluntary – no fee)**
- families concerned with a grandparent's increased frailty contact the health visitor responsible for the care of elderly people **(NHS – no fee)**
- parents of an adult with severe learning disabilities contact a private residential care home **(private – fee involved)**.

Referral by emergency services

In the case of referral by emergency services this involves clients in a crisis situation. This may be through the National Health Service, or local services. Local services vary according to the locality in which people live, and refer to services other than those provided by the NHS. They are local authorities in England, Scotland and Wales, and health and social care authorities in Northern Ireland.

You need to understand what emergency local services are available in your area. Examples of referral by emergency services include:

- casualties from a road accident are taken to a hospital accident and emergency department **(NHS – no charge)**

- an adult has a mild heart attack requiring the attention of a GP **(NHS – free treatment, possible prescription fee)**, possibly followed by a **professional referral** to a cardiac specialist

- a young person suddenly displays excessively eccentric, self-damaging behaviour. Friends phone the police – **referral by others** – who contact the local psychiatric hospital **(NHS – no fee)**

- a parent is arrested and imprisoned. The partner is in shock and incapable of caring for their small children. Social services find accommodation and provide care for the children and partner **(local service – no fee)**.

ACTIVITY 5

Work out and record in a suitable format which organisation in your own locality would deal with the four emergencies described here.

Performance Criterion 4

Support for Client Groups to Make Use of Services

Support for client groups to make use of services includes information about services and how to access them, and about rights within services, the use of a translator and the use of an advocate.

Information about services and how to access them

(see also Unit 1, Element 2)

A service is of little use if no one knows anything about it. Information can be provided in a variety of ways:

- paper based – books

    – posters

    – leaflets, etc.

- on audiotapes

- on radio

- on video or television

- word of mouth – formally, in schools, colleges or lectures

    – informally, from friends and family.

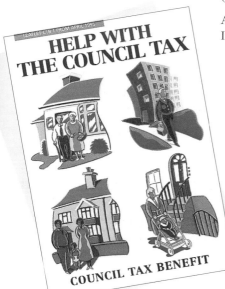

unit three

The method of presentation is vitally important, and must be appropriate for the target group.

The following lists examples where appropriateness is important.

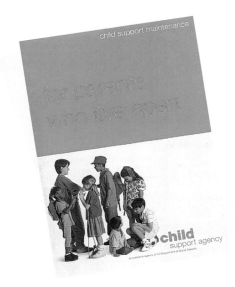

- A small percentage of elderly people in the UK have HIV. Information on support and how to access it must be presented differently from that targeting young gay people.

- Young people in mainstream education need information on where they can have access to counselling. So do young people in a nearby school for students with moderate learning disabilities. The information needs presenting differently for each group.

- Visually-impaired women have right of access to well-women clinics. It would not be appropriate to give this information visually in the same way as publicity aimed at sighted women.

- Individuals who do not use English as a first language need information in their own language and dialect. They also need access to health and social care workers who understand their culture and can pass on information sympathetically and realistically.

ACTIVITY 6

1 List the places where you have seen information on health and social care services displayed.

2 What form did it take?

3 Do you think it was accessible to most of the public?

4 Do you think it would appeal to most of the public?

5 Was it understandable to those who would see it?

6 Record your information, mentioning percentages and ratios where you consider it appropriate. **[NUM 2.2]**

Information about rights within services

All clients have a right to

- **access to services**

- **confidentiality** – no information gained about them in the course of services being delivered must be shared outside the professional setting (see also Unit 4, Element 3)

- **non-discriminatory treatment** – in the United Kingdom all clients are entitled to equal treatment, access to services, and quality of care. This is stated in all written policies connected with the health and social care services, the Patients' Charter and the Community Care Charter. This means that no one should be

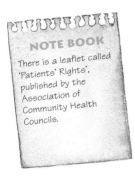

discriminated against because they are of a different race or culture, or have different beliefs from the majority of the population. Males and females should be treated equally. People with disabilities should be on equal footing with able-bodied people. An individual's age should not be held against them. In short, everyone should be treated in the same way. (See also Unit 4, Element 2.)

Use of a translator

All clients have the right to be understood and to understand.

This includes individuals who:

- do not speak or understand English fluently
- are deaf and communicate through British Sign Language or in other ways
- have physical or learning disabilities which prevent them from understanding or speaking easily.

Where a client uses a service in a neighbourhood where their own language is not commonly used, they are entitled to the help of a translator if necessary. Others with communication problems are also entitled to help from someone who is used to their own way of 'speaking'.

Use of an advocate

An advocate is someone who responds on behalf of another person who is unable to act for him or herself. This is different from the service given by a translator, who interprets only someone else's spoken thoughts and wishes. Some areas have set up Citizen Advocacy Systems, which work especially in the area of mental health and with clients who are disadvantaged or have learning difficulties. Currently there are plans to extend this into a National Advocacy Network.

unit three

Advocacy is about
- Helping people to speak up for themselves or speaking on their behalf if necessary
- Helping people to become involved in their own care and to become independent as possible. This is called **self-advocacy** and **empowers** people.
- Ensuring that rights and choices are respected, and helping those who are disadvantaged or who have disabilities to participate as fully as possible in society.
- Making sure that the client has equal power with the service providers.
- Forming partnerships between client and advocate so that one can speak for the other in an impartial way in an atmosphere of trust and confidence.

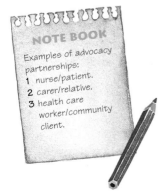

Case Studies

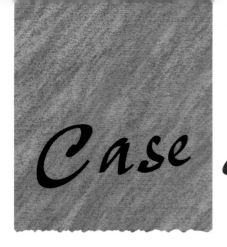

Case study 1   Netherfield Comunity Care *(Continued from Element 3.1)*

Horace is chatting to Debbie in his house. He is sharing his fears of losing his independence. Debbie is reassuring him that his family and Mikhail are working together to help him to stay at home for the foreseeable future, despite the fact that his sight is failing and he is increasingly bewildered by the pace of life, especially when, as now, he feels threatened. As his family live in another county, Horace cannot understand how they managed to contact the Netherfield team.

Task 1

1   How might Debbie explain to Horace the different ways in which his family might have gained access to his local services?

2   What services might Netherfield provide for people in Horace's situation?

Task 1

3   What support could be provided to help Horace to make informed choices from the services Netherfield can provide?

Case study 2   Hill Hall
(Continued from Element 3.1)

Molly is describing to Ann how some of the clients came to be admitted to the school. The most memorable occasion occurred when Roberta's mother left her on the doorstep one morning when she was seven years old, because she felt she could no longer cope with her severe disabilities on her own at home. More usually the children are referred from professionals.

Task 2

1   Using the information from pc3, consider

   a   Freddie, whose parents took him first to their GP at the age of two, when the family returned from living abroad

   b   Rumi, whose learning difficulties were first noticed at the local health care clinic

Task 2

   c   Roberta, described on the left.

2   Make a flow diagram to illustrate the route taken for each of the clients, identifying each method of referral used to gain support from Hill Hall.

Task 2

3   Remembering Usha, the Asian girl who attends Hill Hall, describe the support which she and her family may have received to help them to make best use of Hill Hall's local services.

Case study 3   The Thatched Cottage

(Continued from Element 3.1)

Dora and Mark are discussing the new facilities. Mark imagines that most of the new clients will come from private homes, but Dora says that Brian is recovering from a recent stroke and has not long been out of hospital, and Ada is visiting regularly from a local NHS long-stay hospital which is closing down. She may be transferring to The Thatched Cottage if she likes it there. Maggie, acting on a suggestion by her chapel minister, comes to be with her husband, who is a permanent resident as he has had both legs amputated.

Task 1

1   Work out how Brian, Ada and Maggie might have been referred for day care in The Thatched Cottage.

2   What might be Brian and Ada's needs? Which NHS services might be addressing those needs?

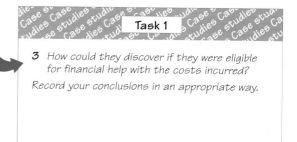

Task 1

3   How could they discover if they were eligible for financial help with the costs incurred?

Record your conclusions in an appropriate way.

Case study 4   Down Way School

(Continued from Element 3.1)

Having produced their booklet to help new parents to find out local sources of help and support, Jalwinder and Isabel decide to see how useful it has been. They select some parents to chat with when they bring their children to school to see which of the services chosen by Jalwinder have actually been useful. They choose Mr Sanderson, a widower who works full time, Mrs Wong, who has no transport and a toddler to care for as well as Andrew, who is in the reception class, and Bob Green, who is bringing up his children alone on a limited income.

Task 1

1   Which of the organisations described by Jalwinder in her booklet might be useful to the three families described above?

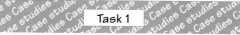

Task 1

2   How could the families find out about their rights within any of the services they might choose to use?

3   Where could they find such information?

unit three case studies

Multiple Choice Questions

1 Which of the following methods of referral to services is *most* accurately described as referral by a non-health professional?

    a advised by clergyman

    b recommended by GP

    c referred by health visitor

    d contacted by relative

2 An advocate is someone who

    a takes over from clients

    b admits clients to care

    c helps clients to help themselves

    d interprets for clients

3 Dysfunction means

    a not working properly

    b disease is present

    c emotionally disturbed

    d motor disability

4 Which of the following means the same as the phrase 'learning difficulties'?

    a learning disabilities

    b schizophrenia

    c motor impairment

    d mental health problems

5 An acute disease is one which is

    a severe

    b temporary

    c incurable

    d permanent

6 Congenital disabilities are the result of

    a hormone deficiency

    b genetic inheritance

    c acquired trauma

    d sensory deprivation

7 Accessing services means

    a providing ramps and lifts in buildings

    b making care provision easily available

    c making professional referral straightforward

    d providing services free at the point of delivery

8 Clients with acute physical needs are *most* likely to need

    a physiotherapy

    b short term care

    c informal support

    d long term care

9 Which of the following *best* describes the use of advocates?

    a a way of helping clients to make use of services

    b a method of referral to services

    c referral to local authority provision

    d a way of accessing emergency service

Summary of Evidence Opportunities and Their Relationship to Performance Criteria

Activities 1, 2 and 3	pc 1	**Activity 6**	pc 4	**Case study 4**	pcs 2 and 4
Activity 4	pc 2	**Case study 1**	pcs all		
Activity 5	pc 3	**Case studies 2 and 3**	pcs 3 and 4		

Unit 3 Element 2 Summary of Element Range and Personal Evidence Tracking Record

Element range references (tick against left-hand column)	Description of evidence	Pc and range covered	Portfolio reference number
Pc 1 Needs			
physical – acute			
– chronic			
emotional			
mental			
social			
Client groups			
babies			
children			
young people			
adults			
elderly people			
families			
Pc 2 Services provided			
free at the point of delivery			
for which a basic fee may need to be paid			
ability to pay taken into account			
run on a charitable basis			
for which the individual pays			
by the family or local community			
Pc 3 Methods of referral			
professional referral			
self-referral			
referral by others			
emergency services			
– NHS			
– local services			

unit three

Unit 3 Element 2 Summary of Element Range and Personal Evidence Tracking Record			
Element range references *(tick against left-hand column)*	**Description of evidence**	**Pc and range covered**	**Portfolio reference number**
Pc 4 Support			
information			
– about services			
– how to access			
– about rights within services			
translators			
advocates			

Element 3.3

Investigate Jobs in Health and Social Care

Performance Criteria

pc 1 Identify the main jobs in health and social care services — 159

pc 2 Describe the day-to-day work of people with jobs in health and social care — 163

pc 3 Describe the career routes of people with jobs in health and social care — 164

pc 4 Compare the actual role of people who work in health and social care with stereotypes of those roles — 166

Summary of evidence opportunities and their relationship to the pcs — 171

Summary of element range and personal evidence tracking record — 171

Introduction

In the last element we examined clients. Now we look at those who work with them, who are commonly called **carers**. This word covers the numerous jobs in the care field, including health care workers, social workers, and those supporting them by effective administration.

The everyday work of carers is described, along with the qualifications needed to move into jobs. Lastly we look at our perceptions of what is involved in these jobs, and compare them with the reality of the working life of a carer.

Performance Criterion 1

The Main Jobs in Health and Social Care Services

The health and social services are very much intertwined. Together they cover the **provision of care** and **support services**. We will be looking at jobs in the National Health Service, local authorities, including education, the private sector, the voluntary sector, and informal care provided by the family and local community.

unit three

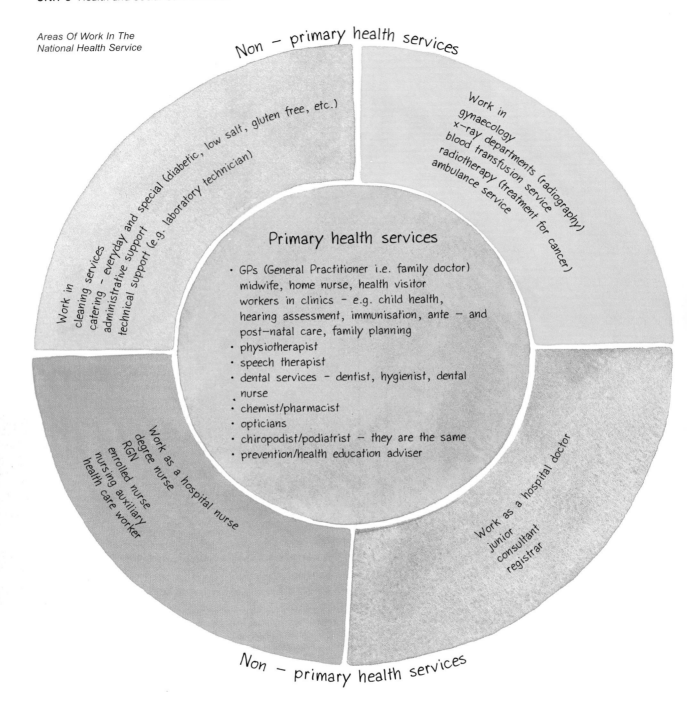

Non – primary health services

Work in
gymaecology
x-ray departments (radiography)
blood transfusion service
radiotherapy (treatment for cancer)
ambulance service

Work in
cleaning services
catering – everyday and special (diabetic, low salt, gluten free, etc.)
administrative support
technical support (e.g. laboratory technician)

Primary health services

- GPs (General Practitioner i.e. family doctor)
  midwife, home nurse, health visitor
  workers in clinics – e.g. child health,
  hearing assessment, immunisation, ante – and
  post–natal care, family planning
- physiotherapist
- speech therapist
- dental services – dentist, hygienist, dental
  nurse
- chemist/pharmacist
- opticians
- chiropodist/podiatrist – they are the same
- prevention/health education adviser

Work as a hospital nurse
degree nurse
RGN
enrolled nurse
nursing auxiliary
health care worker

Work as a hospital doctor
junior
consultant
registrar

Non – primary health services

The National Health Service

The diagram above describes the areas of work in the National Health
Service.

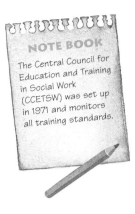

NOTE BOOK

The Central Council for Education and Training in Social Work (CCETSW) was set up in 1971 and monitors all training standards.

Local authorities

Social services

In the provision of social care, carers often work as

- caseworkers (with specific cases)
- fieldworkers (regularly working with specific clients)
- community workers (in the community with specific groups)

although these roles overlap.

Social workers are able to bring the statutory and voluntary services together to meet the immediate needs of people in times of crisis, and report in a practical way on how the services work together and with clients.

The table below describes areas of work within the social services.

Areas Of Work In Social Services

Residential care

residential care worker
management of residential homes
registration and inspection of social care establishments
organising volunteers
statistics, publicity, etc.
expenditure control

Social work

social work services outside residential care
family placement of children needing care
court/school/police liaison
GP practice and hospital social workers
children - child protection, family work secure units etc.
services for disabled people – e.g. visually impaired
services for disadvantaged people – e.g. homeless
community work

Domiciliary services

home help
day nurseries, day centres
aids and adaptations for disabled people to use at home.
luncheon clubs
'Meals on Wheels'
adult training centres
rehabilitation centres i.e. helping people to become independent

Management

salaries and wages
recruitment
secretarial services
supplies
collection contributions towards care where appropriate
burial arrangements (if there are no family of friends)
training, assessment, and provision

Areas of work in education

Education

Jobs
teacher
classroom assistant (non-teaching)
technician
head teacher
bursar (looks after funds)
secretarial work
administration
caterer
cleaner
gardener
buildings supervisor/caretaker

Age groups	Sector
nurseries	state, private, voluntary
infant/junior/primary	state, private, voluntary, grant maintained
secondary	state, private, grant maintained
further education higher education adult education	all are independent of local authority control

Grant maintained means that the school manages its own budget with money provided by the state

unit three

The voluntary sector

Examples of services provided by the voluntary sector include Dr Barnados, MIND, and The Samaritans. Most of their workers are volunteers and are unpaid. They may or may not be trained. Larger organisations need salaried staff with professional training to manage them.

Those who want to volunteer for work with a charitable organisation need to contact the Citizens Advice Bureau or their local Social Services Department. Training may or may not be part of the package. Sometimes a first aid qualification is required; sometimes, as in the area of counselling, specific training is demanded.

People's motives for working as volunteers are as varied as those of all carers. To some it is a sense of duty or a religious commitment which leads them to the work, others see it as an antidote to the boredom of retirement or unemployment.

Others have skills they want to share. Some use voluntary work to gain practical experience for paid occupation. There are those that wish to add weight to a pressure group for reform, and some who become involved out of sheer goodwill and gratitude for personal good fortune.

The private and self-employed sector

The private and self-employed sector provides services such as residential day care, child care, health care and other services such as laundry.

Areas of work in the private sector

Residential and day care	Services
proprietor/owner/manager	laundry
RGN (Registered General Nurse)	cleaning
enrolled nurse	hairdressing
care assistant	chiropody/podiatry
respite care	occupational therapy
'sitting' schemes (relieving carers in their homes)	physiotherapy

Child care	Health care
play groups – owner	occupational therapy
manager	chiropody/podiatry
assistant	dentistry
holiday companies and tour operators	physiotherapy
nanny	alternative medicine
childminder	homeopathy
foster parent	reflexology
	acupuncture
	aromatherapy
	chiropractic
	osteopathy

Informal care

Most health and social care is carried out by ordinary people within their families, or by specialist local groups.

One of the aims of the Community Care Act is that people should remain as independent as possible in their own homes. Thus the role of health and care social workers within the community has taken on a new and important significance. It is part of their role to work with informal carers and to link them with services which might make life easier for all concerned.

Performance Criterion 2

The Day-To-Day Work of People With Jobs in Health and Social Care

In studying people's work in the health and social care field, we will be examining work patterns, working with client groups, and hours of work.

Work patterns

Work patterns vary within the areas of health and social care and the following list gives the main types of working patterns:

- alone – childminders, foster parents

- in teams with the same discipline – a dental practice with a dentist, dental nurse and hygienist

- in teams of people from other disciplines but with similar goals

    – GP's practice with a GP, practice nurse, community nurse, health visitor, chiropodist

    – community mental health team of social workers, community psychiatric nurse, clinical psychologist, community worker.

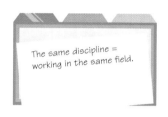

The same discipline = working in the same field.

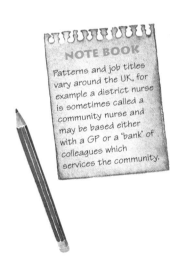

NOTE BOOK

Patterns and job titles vary around the UK, for example a district nurse is sometimes called a community nurse and may be based either with a GP or a 'bank' of colleagues which services the community.

Working with client groups

Those who have a close working relationship with clients can be regarded as being involved with treatment, enablement, or a combination of these two.

Treatment is the easier to define. It refers to the carer who is actively involved with caring for the physical or mental health of a client.

Enablement literally means making someone more able. Thus a social worker will make a client *more able* to be independent. A physiotherapist makes a client *more able* to move freely. An occupational therapist makes people *more able* to manipulate things and use their surrounding effectively.

Hours of work

Those working in the care services have work hours which vary greatly. Many workers are attracted by the unpredictability of the job and the irregular hours, feeling that they would find 'nine-to-five' work monotonous.

Some carers work during the day-time, others at night. This can be a matter of choice, or something imposed by the needs of clients. Both day and night work can be regular, or arranged into varying **shifts**.

Holiday time varies from job to job, but many carers work at Christmas and other times when many people are on holiday.

unit three

Performance Criterion 3

The Career Routes of People with Jobs in Health and Social Care

Consideration of career routes needs to include study of qualifications and other entry requirements, previous jobs and possible future jobs, and opportunities for job relocation. These five aspects are covered together in the following text.

Qualifications to enter

These can be either

vocational, e.g. NVQs, first aid certificates, work-based training, and are

- practical, preparing for the world of work
- skills-based with background knowledge
- gained through training or work experience.

GNVQs are at present included in the vocational category – those at Advanced level are sometimes referred to as 'vocational A levels'.

Or

academic, e.g. GCSE, A levels, degrees, diplomas, and are

- knowledge based
- gained through school/college/university, or by independent study linked to a college or university base.

To work in the field of health and social care or education, you need to decide how much you enjoy working close to people. If you like company, and relate well to others, you may choose a job which involves direct contact with clients. If you want to help society but are not enthusiastic about interacting with individuals needing care, you may prefer to go into the administrative, technical or support side of health or social care.

National Vocational Qualifications (NVQs)

Until recently the majority of workers in the UK had no nationally recognised qualification. To put this right, the NVQs were devised; they are awarded for skills and competence in a working situation.

The field of health and social care has been included in this revolutionary process. The NVQs in Care are designed for those working in residential and day care. The NVQs in Child Care and Education are for those looking after children up to seven years of age. There are NVQs in Operating Theatre Practice, Neurophysiology, Criminal Justice Services, Catering and Hospitality and other areas in the field of health and social care.

Although the NVQs are primarily intended to reward **skills**, as they proceed up through the levels the **knowledge content** becomes more significant.

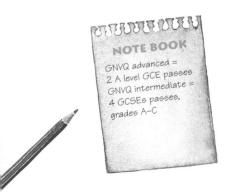

NOTE BOOK
GNVQ advanced =
2 A level GCE passes
GNVQ intermediate =
4 GCSEs passes,
grades A–C

General National Vocational Qualifications (GNVQs)

The GNVQs are, unlike the NVQs, knowledge-based, and are currently mainly gained in schools and colleges. Their method of assessment (by various ways of providing evidence) has evolved from the NVQ systems.

Routes to jobs

GNVQ Intermediate	Degree	Vocational
+ NVQ care assistant, health care worker, community care worker child care **+ GNVQ Advanced** **+ A Level** – nursing **+ A level** – teaching *(varies according to locality)*	*via A level, GNVQ Advanced or a mix of both* Junior doctor, registrar, GP, surgeon, consultant some nursing; general or psychiatric, midwifery, health visiting, specialist nurse social work administration dentistry teaching health promotion pharmacy management physiotherapy	some nursing; general or psychiatric, midwifery, health visiting, specialist nurse ambulance service cleaning services home help management nursing auxiliary health care worker community care worker care assistant classroom assistant secretarial work teaching

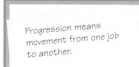

Progression means movement from one job to another.

General notes on work in the care field

Routes to jobs are becoming more flexible, making change and progression easier. Mature employees often have their experience taken into consideration. A woman who has been a classroom assistant while her family was young may find it easy to make a career change through teacher training if she meets the academic requirements. Or an experienced health care worker with a level 3 in NVQ in Care may be accepted for nurse training if other requirements are also met.

Some jobs and qualifications give access to work throughout the UK, others are more localised. Nurses are needed everywhere, while other work is clustered more in some areas than others. For instance, more social workers are needed in inner city areas than rural ones.

Some jobs in care have a minimum age requirement. Social workers have to be 21.

The diagram above outlines the various routes to jobs in health and social care.

unit three

Performance Criterion 4

The Actual Role of People who Work in Health and Social Care Compared with Stereotypes of These Roles

Before coming face-to-face with the realities of what is actually involved in the everyday work of someone in the care field, we all have our ideas of what their job might entail. We are given visual and verbal pictures of stereotypical images of many workers.

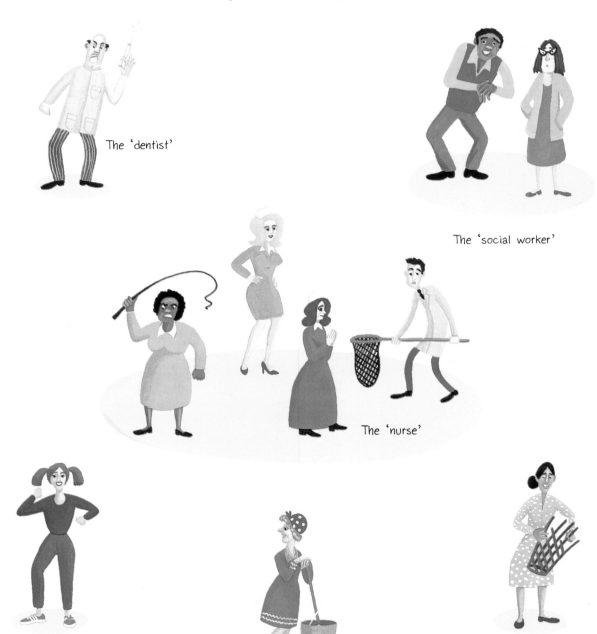

The 'dentist'

The 'social worker'

The 'nurse'

The 'physiotherapist'

The 'home help'

The 'occupational therapist'

Florence Nightingale's job did not entail her gliding endlessly around darkened wards with her candle, while adoring soldiers kissed her shadow. She was more likely to have had to tuck her skirts up to avoid the mud and slime, and the wards would have been full of dreadful smells, blood-soaked dressings and emotionally scarred patients.

So we need to examine in a realistic way the actualities of care work, realising that part of its attraction is that it is full of endless variety arising from many different aspects of humanity.

Some aspects of care work

Pay (*approx*)

staff nurse £10–£12,000 pa
sister £13–19,000 pa
health care assistant £7–9,000 pa
care assistant £154.35 pw
ward secretary *from* £6,000 pa
social worker £11–18,000 pa
community care worker £7–9,000
education welfare officer £11-18,000 pa
dentist £36,000+ pa
dental nurse £95–165 pw
hygienist £10–11,000 pa
radiographer £12–14,000 pa
occupational therapist £12–14,000 pa
health service manager £8–33,000 pa
medical records clerk £7–8,000 pa
medical secretary *from* £8,500 pa
ambulance person £9–14,000 pa
teacher £11–31,000 pa
school technician £5–9,000 pa
classroom assistant £160 pw

pa = per annum pw = per week
Source: Careers and Occupational Information Centre 1994

Working conditions

staff room
rest room
meal times
hours on standby
shifts/rotas
training possibilities
opportunities for travel
opportunities for career moves
within the UK
'strokes' (see Notebook)
resources

Work place

hospital ward
community
clinic
nursing homes
care homes
office
people's homes
community
schools

Main Tasks

administration
report writing
training others
treatments
dressings
toileting
washing
feeding
family work
counselling
record keeping
guidance
listening
giving medicines
attending meetings
advocacy
telephoning
meeting the public
liaising

unit three

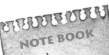

NOTE BOOK

'Strokes'
When someone is nice to you, it is said that you are 'receiving strokes' which make you feel good. For many in the nursing field,

it is these 'strokes' from patients that make up for long hours and unpleasant tasks; they are a reward not measured in financial terms.
In some areas of care, clients pass on a lot of 'strokes' which reduce stress.

In other areas the 'stokes' are few, and do little to counteract the stresses from long hours, paperwork demands, and time-consuming requests which seem to be unrelated to the work in hand.

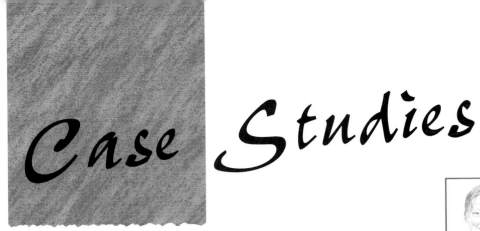

Case Studies

Case study 1   Netherfield Community Care

(Continued from Element 3.2)

While she and Mikhail have been working with Horace and his family, Debbie has been amazed at the variety of care workers who are becoming involved with the case. She has had a vague ambition to become a 'social worker', but now realises that it could be unrealistic for her to aim for a career requiring a degree, and decides to explore other avenues to community work. She asks Mikhail where she can find accurate, up-to-date information about jobs in health and social care in Netherfield. He brings her a list describing the various areas of work.

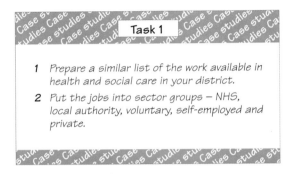

Task 1

1   Prepare a similar list of the work available in health and social care in your district.

2   Put the jobs into sector groups – NHS, local authority, voluntary, self-employed and private.

Case study 2   Hill Hall

(continued from Element 3.2)

In a tutorial session, the students are comparing notes about their work experience. Debbie and Ann are talking about their plans for the future. Ann, although more accepting of the emotional stress of caring, still feels a bit nervous of tasks involving intimate and personal care of clients. But she dislikes the idea of routine office work, and wishes to commit herself to the care services. Debbie brings out Mikhail's list and shares it with the group. Together they work out jobs which Ann and others who share her feelings might undertake.

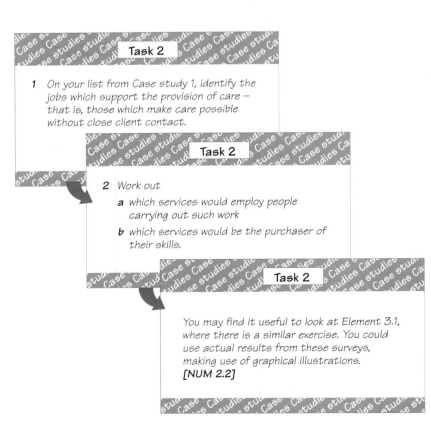

Task 2

1   On your list from Case study 1, identify the jobs which support the provision of care – that is, those which make care possible without close client contact.

Task 2

2   Work out

a   which services would employ people carrying out such work

b   which services would be the purchaser of their skills.

Task 2

You may find it useful to look at Element 3.1, where there is a similar exercise. You could use actual results from these surveys, making use of graphical illustrations. **[NUM 2.2]**

Case study 3   The Thatched Cottage

Before he started working at The Thatched Cottage, Mark had wanted to go to a psychiatric hospital for his work experience, but he was too young. However, he now enjoys his placement. He expected it to be boring, but has found that he was mistaken. The residents have become real people to him. By the time they were his age, some had lived through the First World War, and their conversations are far from tedious. He likes the residents who are confused or demented most, as they come closest to his dream of working in mental health.

Task 3

1 How has Mark's idea of working in residential care for the elderly changed as he has become involved? What factors might have caused him to change his mind?

2 In what way will his experience be valuable if he pursues his ambition to be a mental health care worker?

Task 3

3 If Mark lived in your area, what choices would be open to him in the field of mental health?

4 What skills and qualifications would he need to take up each of the choices?

Record you conclusions in an appropriate format, using Core Skills in an imaginative way.

Case study 4   Down Way School

Adam is six. While he is talking to Jalwinder one day, he tells her that he believes that she, Isabel and all the teaching staff live in the stock cupboard after school finishes each day. He thinks they stand up in line like clothes in a wardrobe. Jalwinder shares this in the staff room one rainy lunchtime, and, after the laughter dies down, the staff begin to discuss misunderstandings they used to hold about adults when they were little, especially about jobs.

Task 4

1 Think about three people known to your group who work as carers
   • one in the support services
   • one in health and medical care
   • one in social care.
   Working in a group, discuss and record what you think each job involves in terms of pay, working conditions and tasks.

Task 4

2 Each word process a letter (including an address label) and send one copy to arrange a meeting with the three people concerned to find out

   • how your image of their work fits in with the reality of their job

Task 4

When dealing with pay structure, use calculations where appropriate. Analysis of average indicators need to be stressed in relevant sections of this case study. **[NUM 2.2]**

3 Compare their responses with your ideas.

4 Word process your conclusions, save on disk and print. **[IT 2.1, 2.2, 2.3]**

Task 4

   • the skills and qualifications they needed before they started

   • if they would recommend their job to a young person starting work

   • whether or not they have received training

   • any ambitions they have for promotion or change of occupation. **[IT 2.1, 2.2, 2.3]**

Multiple Choice Questions

1 A career route is

   a *the way you decide to go to work*

   b *the requirements for entry into a job*

   c *a qualification gained at school or college*

   d *the beginning of work experience*

2 Some of the following statements describe stereotypes of care workers. Which of them gives the *best* reason for becoming a care worker?

   a *all nurses are saints*

   b *everyone who works with psychiatric patients is as crazy as they are*

   c *each carer must choose the work which suits them best*

   d *teachers choose the job because they like the holidays*

3 Which one of the following is a useful interaction with clients?

   a *power*

   b *dependence*

   c *aggression*

   d *enablement*

4 People who wish to take up social work must be

   a *over 18 years old*

   b *under 21 years old*

   c *over 21 years old*

   d *under 30 years old*

5 Which of the following phrases best describes an NVQ?

   a *a vocational award*

   b *a degree*

   c *a GNVQ*

   d *a diploma*

6 Which of the following is an example of a team of the same discipline?

   a *a classroom assistant, a care assistant, an enrolled nurse*

   b *a podiatrist (chiropodist), a health care worker, a nanny*

   c *a GP, a Trust hospital, a social worker*

   d *a dentist, a dental nurse, a hygienist*

7 Which of the following *best* describes shift work?

   a *taking turns to work for different periods of time*

   b *frequently moving from one job to another*

   c *working as part of a multidisciplinary team*

   d *having to work with changing client groups*

8 Opportunities for job relocation means

   a *working with a short-term contract*

   b *having to do night duty from time to time*

   c *following a flexible career route*

   d *having the choice to move to similar work elsewhere*

Summary of Evidence Opportunities and Their Relationship to Performance Criteria

Activity 1	pc 1	**Case study 3**	pcs 3 and 4
Case study 1	pc 1 + Elements 3.1, pcs 1 and 2	**Case study 4**	pcs 2, 3 and 4
Case study 2	pc 1 + Element 3.1, pc 1		

Unit 3 Element 3 Summary of Element Range and Personal Evidence Tracking Record

Element range references *(tick against left-hand column)*	Description of evidence	Pc and range covered	Portfolio reference number
Pc 1 Jobs			
provision of care			
support services			
Pc 2 Work			
work patterns			
– alone			
– in a team of the same discipline			
– in a team from other disciplines			
working with client groups			
– treatment			
– enablement			
hours of work			
– day-time			
– night work			
– shift work			
Pc 3 Career routes			
qualifications			
– vocational			
– academic			
other requirements			
previous jobs			
possible future jobs			
opportunities for job relocation			
Pc 4 Comparison of role with stereotypes			
pay			
working conditions			
tasks			

unit three

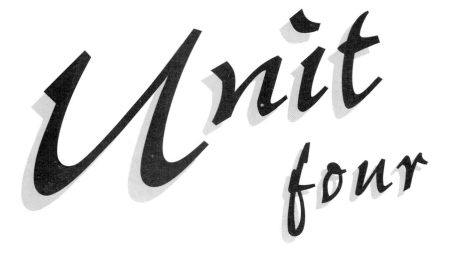

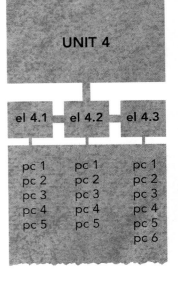

UNIT 4

el 4.1	el 4.2	el 4.3
pc 1	pc 1	pc 1
pc 2	pc 2	pc 2
pc 3	pc 3	pc 3
pc 4	pc 4	pc 4
pc 5	pc 5	pc 5
		pc 6

Communication and Inter-Personal Relationships

Elements

4.1 Develop communication skills

4.2 Explore how interpersonal relationships may be affected by discriminatory behaviour

4.3 Investigate aspects of working with clients in health and social care

After you have worked through this unit you will understand why communication and interpersonal relationships need to be effective in health and social care.

In the first element you will be examining your own communication skills to see if they need to be developed to make your relationships with others more meaningful. Self-knowledge and self-evaluation are important for those hoping to work in services in which people are in close contact with others.

The second element explores what happens when people are discriminated against, and how life experiences and cultural influences affect individuals' attitudes.

The third element combines the first two in looking at issues fundamental to interpersonal relationships in health and social care, such as confidentiality and the nature of client/carer relationships.

You will find that this unit relates to Unit 2, especially Elements 2.2 and 2.3, and also that it is particularly relevant to communication core skills.

Effective = useful and purposeful.

Fundamental = forming foundations.

Element 4.1

Develop Communication Skills

Performance Criteria

pc 1 Explain why it is important for individuals, families, and groups to communicate — 173

pc 2 Demonstrate listening and responding skills to encourage communication with individuals in different contexts — 177

pc 3 Demonstrate observation skills to encourage communication with individuals in different contexts — 181

pc 4 Identify obstacles to effective communication — 182

pc 5 Evaluate one's own communication skills and make suggestions for their improvement — 185

Summary of evidence opportunities and their relationship to the pcs — 191

Summary of element range and personal evidence tracking record — 191

Introduction

When we **communicate** we are in touch with another person or a group, and sharing, exchanging or passing on information. From infancy to old age we communicate with the world around us – we may even talk to ourselves frequently !

Communication brings **power**. Good communicators can adjust what they say and how they say it to ensure that those receiving their information understand it. So they will subtly change their vocabulary, their accent, or their body language to make the listener feel at ease and more likely to listen to what is being said.

Power brings responsibility. A carer who is a good communicator will use the power which follows to inform, encourage, reassure and help clients. Good communication skills are used irresponsibly when they are deployed to manipulate, bully or intimidate other people.

Performance Criterion 1

The Importance of Communication for Individuals, Families and Groups

We will be looking at the role of communication in intellectual, emotional and social development of the individual, personal beliefs and preferences (including culture, religion, politics, sexuality), and development of groups.

Speaking and listening are difficult if there is anything wrong with the mouth, tongue and vocal cords, or with the ears. Equally important is the state of development of the brain, where messages are received

unit four

and understood. This is why children with physical disabilities may have problems with communication.

Development of self

Half of children's mental capacity will have developed before they are four. Learning is much faster if the child has language skills. Thoughts, feelings, ideas and attitudes are easier to grasp through words. Reading extends our horizons. Discussion helps to form our ideas. Listening puts us in touch with other people's views. Thus our powers of communication extend our knowledge and help our intelligence to develop.

Intellectual development

Babies learn to speak as their muscles and systems develop and their understanding matures. In their pre-verbal stage babies cry, smile, gurgle, and make eye contact to communicate with their carers. Infants 'scribble talk' and babble and from 9 months they may say simple words.

People with learning difficulties or physical disabilities may never be able to speak clearly or use a wide vocabulary. If their eye–hand co-ordination is adequate they may be able to use a word board or a word processor, or point to pictures. Communication like this is slow and can lead to frustration unless the client is helped with patience and sensitivity. Many clients exceed everybody's predictions about their abilities if they are surrounded by encouraging and supportive carers.

Social and emotional development

As children grow up they learn to behave in a manner which is acceptable to the people around them. Their personalities usually develop within the family. Their responses to the family's behaviour determines how their emotions develop. Children whose social and emotional development has been hampered by social or emotional deprivations are often poor communicators.

Personal beliefs and preferences

As we grow and our ability to communicate by receiving and interpreting information develops, we begin to find out who we are, and to decide what our personal beliefs and preferences will be.

If someone has not had much contact with the outside world, individual choices may have been very narrow. This is why infant schools and nurseries try to provide as wide a spread of experiences as possible to children who may not have a range of possibilities at home. Carers often provide **guided choice**, which means that clients' choice is limited to, say, five options to avoid muddle and confusion.

To decide on personal beliefs and preferences people need to be able to exchange views and information about how they feel. Some people adopt their families' beliefs which have surrounded them since

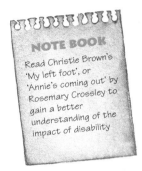

NOTE BOOK

Read Christie Brown's 'My left foot', or 'Annie's coming out' by Rosemary Crossley to gain a better understanding of the impact of disability

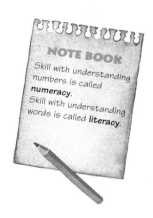

NOTE BOOK

Skill with understanding numbers is called **numeracy**.
Skill with understanding words is called **literacy**.

ACTIVITY 1

1 Record socially acceptable gestures and symbols.

2 Explain why they are effective.

infancy, which is why culture and religious traditions survive for generations, and why children may copy their parents' job choices and lifestyles. If children feel the need to turn their backs on their families' ways, good communication with parents can make this a friendly experience, while without good communication family splits and hostilities may occur. The social and emotional development of those with language and speech impairment is affected by teasing and mimicry, so that they feel rejected and isolated. People who are autistic do not appreciate jokes and high spirits, which is difficult for society to understand and causes them to feel rejected.

Young people especially like to talk to each other at great length, in school or college, at clubs and pubs. In adolescence, the foundations of adulthood are forming, so talking about things helps to consolidate feelings and ease anxieties. Lonely young people find this time especially hard if they have no friends in which to confide about everything from family relationships through to politics and sexuality.

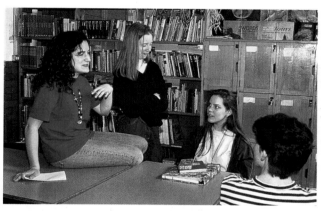

The social development of children with sensory impairment is often problematical. They find it hard to interpret other people's actions. Visually impaired people find it hard to learn by copying other people – a major factor in our social development – and cannot receive non-verbal messages like facial expressions and body language. They run the risk of offending by using inappropriate gestures, and will need to be taught socially acceptable way of using non-verbal communications.

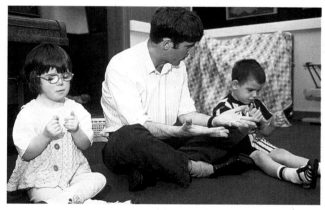

We acquire our concepts of the world mainly through spoken language. Hearing impaired people find it hard to describe ideas or to understand feelings. They may appear to be slow learners, especially if their hearing problems are late in being identified, and their social development is often delayed as others find them hard to relate to, which in turn can cause difficulties with emotional development.

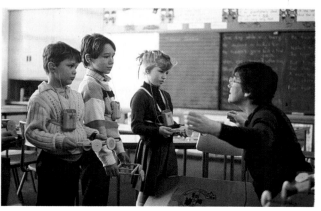

unit four

Development of groups and families

The importance of communication to social interaction

In Unit 2 we looked at the development of relationships. Now we need to see what part communication has to play in this.

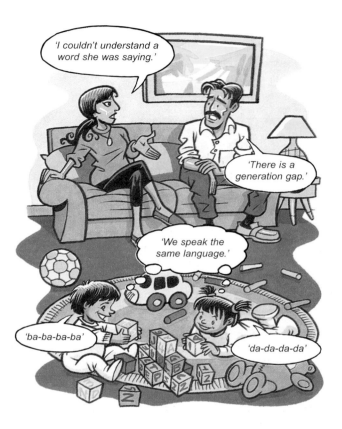

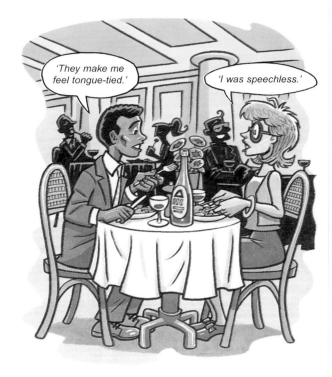

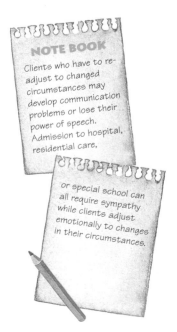

Communication with others is a basic human need. Children who have been actively encouraged to communicate find it natural to share experiences, co-operate with others, work out the results of their actions, make comparisons and share their feelings. This gives them an advantage as emotionally secure adults, able to think and reason, understand and sympathise, and to share all of these by effective communication.

Conversely, some clients have few of these advantages, and need to be persuaded and encouraged to share their true feelings so that they can be helped in the best possible way.

The **language of emotions** is rich, and uses rare words which may not be easily understood; words like 'distress', 'anxiety', 'foreboding', 'dread', 'depression', 'elation', 'apprehension', 'pain', 'excitement', 'pleasure', 'admiration', and 'hope'. When peoples' emotional vocabulary is limited to 'love', as in 'I love that song' or hate, as in 'I hate that food', it is hard for them to convey accurately how they feel when it really matters. They need practice before they can express exactly what their emotional needs are.

Performance Criterion 2

Listening and Responding Skills to Encourage Communication with Individuals in Different Contexts

We communicate in many different ways. These include

- facial expression
- body language and eye contact
- sensory contact – that is, touch
- posture
- prompts, paraphrasing and summarising
- asking open and closed questions
- the tone, pitch and pace of our communication.

These seven methods are covered together within the text which follows.

Communicating effectively requires a combination of verbal and non-verbal methods. We may learn as much by looking as we do by listening, which is why some people prefer meeting face to face to speaking on the telephone. The table below lists what you can do to help clients with language.

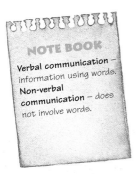

NOTE BOOK
Verbal communication – information using words.
Non-verbal communication – does not involve words.

Helping clients with language

• Talk and listen, with much eye contact.	• Go to the library together.
• Play/work together.	• Keep a scrap book.
• Read stories, watch and discuss TV programmes together.	• Play with blowing bubbles, sucking a ping pong ball on a straw.
• Bathe the client in language. Give a running commentary about whatever you or they happen to be doing.	• Remember that it takes about a year of listening to a language before children can speak it.
• Use language that can be understood.	• Use pauses as a clue that it is the client's turn to speak.
• Introduce to many new experiences and objects.	
• Show that you value their opinion.	
• Give them books, even if reading is hard. Make them age-appropriate, not babyish, and match their interests e.g. football, pop music.	

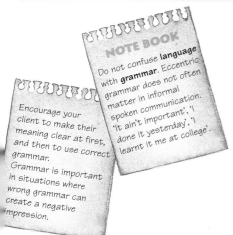

NOTE BOOK
Do not confuse language with **grammar**. Eccentric grammar does not often matter in informal spoken communication. 'It ain't important', 'I done it yesterday', 'I learnt it me at college'.

Encourage your client to make their meaning clear at first, and then to use correct grammar. Grammar is important in situations where wrong grammar can create a negative impression.

Appropriate facial expressions, body language, eye contact and posture

We need to make sure our facial expressions and body language are not giving a wrong message to the person speaking to us. If we begin to register disapproval before someone has finished telling us something important, he or she could alter what is being said to fit what he or she guessed we were thinking.

This often matters less in an informal situation that it does in a formal one, because when people feel relaxed enough to be totally honest with one another it is easier to put misunderstandings right later.

unit four

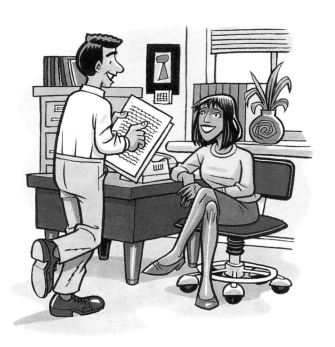

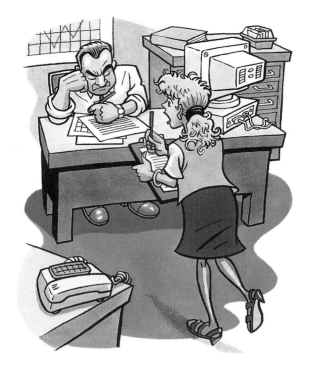

Eye contact implies interest and commitment. Use it even when you think that clients can neither see nor appreciate it – maybe because of impaired vision or confusion. Don't automatically expect eye contact from clients. They may be unaware of its importance or not interested in it, or unable to achieve it because of physical incapacity. Talk about the importance of eye contact to clients if it falls within your role in the workplace.

Posture

Most of what we communicate is conveyed in a way other than speech. Try lowering the volume on the television and see if you can guess what is going on from people's posture and body language. Think about pets. They manage to let us know a great deal without saying a word: 'I want feeding'; 'I want to go out'; 'I like being with you'; 'Welcome home'.

People give messages from the way they sit, stand, choose their seats in relation to one another, and move their hands, arms and legs. Watch how people unconsciously copy each other. The gestures of the dominant person are often imitated. When listening to clients, carers need to make sure that what they say is matched with how it is being said. They need to behave in a way which shows interest, by nodding, turning towards the speaker, leaning forward a little and sitting in a relaxed yet attentive way. The posture needs to be open, not with the arms folded and legs crossed.

It is important to pick up clues from clients to realise when they are feeling stressed or nervous, such as a tense position, a set expression, shallow breathing, a flushed or pale face, or fidgeting.

ACTIVITY 2

Work out typical postures, body language, facial expressions and eye contact indicating anger, impatience, fear, sympathy, interest and concern.

You could use role play in this activity. Remember to record it in an appropriate way for your portfolio – maybe by video.

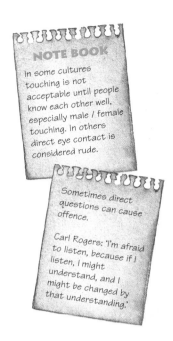

Tips for clear communication

- Speak slowly, using words which are easily understood.
- Make sure people who lip read can see your face – don't stand with the light behind you or cover your mouth with your hand.
- Sit down to talk to people in wheelchairs or in bed, otherwise your body language is saying that you are more important that they are, or that you are anxious to get away.
- Do not talk about important or personal things in busy places. Go somewhere private.
- Seek other people's views. Listen actively.

Warning – don't ask an open question if you only want a short response.

Non-verbal messages are closely linked to acceptable behaviour in the society in which we live. Unlike words, posture and gesture have no fixed meanings and can be misinterpreted. In some societies it is considered unbecoming for a woman to look directly at a man. Smiling to show the teeth is thought to be very rude in some countries. Space is used in different ways. Many British people are most comfortable with a space between them of about two and half feet, and there is generally not much physical contact. Others stand closer together and touch one another more frequently.

Sensory contact

With **confused** people, touch can be misinterpreted as aggression. However, many clients are lonely. Elderly people may have lost a partner, be far from their family, and have had no physical contact for years. When you are sure that your meaning will not be misunderstood and that it is appropriate in the place of work, give your hugs and hand-holding freely, as a means of conveying warmth, sympathy and a willingness to help.

Remember that some people object to being touched. You may need to touch gently people who have **hearing impairment** to catch their attention.

Active listening

To achieve this we need to concentrate to pick out the points of what other people are saying, to try to discover anything underlying the words which they may want to say but do not feel able to. You will get clues from:

- facial expression
- body language and posture
- pauses and noises other than words.
- tone of voice and pitch
- pace of conversation
- choice of words

To do this you need to have distractions at a minimum, be aware of your own prejudices and overcome them, and to be prepared to listen to things you may not want to hear.

The table on the left lists what you can do and what you should avoid doing for clear communication with clients.

When we have conversations, questions help to keep things moving. It is useful to develop skills in selecting the right sort of questions which will encourage the other people to be honest and not put up barriers between their thoughts and the person with whom they are speaking. This involves three main techniques: open questions, closed questions, and prompts.

Open questions

When you ask an **open question** it is like opening a door – they invite long and detailed answers, which will help you to understand people's true meanings. Example of open questions are:

unit four

- 'What's the matter?'

- 'How are you feeling today?'

- Little noises – 'hmm?' 'So?'

- 'How did you get on at the clinic yesterday?'

Closed questions

Closed questions are like closed doors – they invite short answers that may shut the conversation down, because they may only need one-word answers. For example

- 'Tea or coffee?'

- 'Would you like a bath?'

- 'What's your name?'

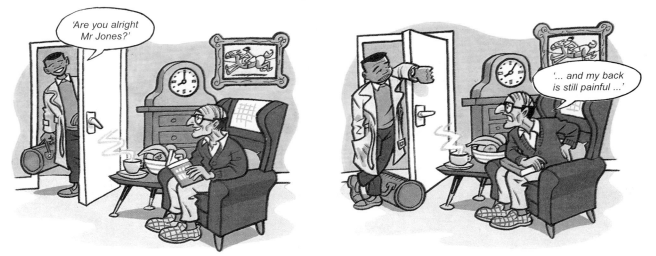

Answer takes five minutes.

or

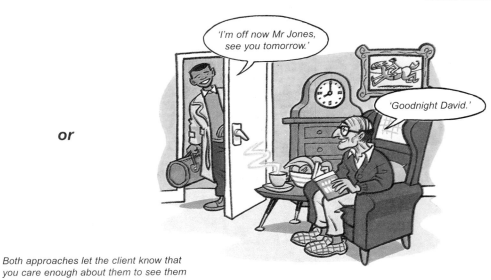

Both approaches let the client know that you care enough about them to see them before going home

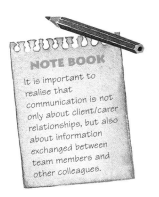

Prompts

Prompts give clues to possible answers. They serve to keep the conversation going. For example

- 'Did you like that?'
- 'Was it difficult?'

Paraphrasing and summarising

We clarify what we think we have heard and understood by statements beginning

- 'Am I right in thinking that you . . . ?'
- 'Do you mean that . . . ?'

This gives the person being spoken to the opportunity to correct any misinterpretation and shows that you have been listening and therefore that you care.

Tone, pitch and pace of communication

When talking to a client, you need to consider the impact of your

- **tone** - for example, loud, angry or sympathetic
- **pitch** - for example, simple and clear for young children, or using longer and more complicated sentences for a more mature person
- **pace** - fast or slow.

Performance Criterion 3

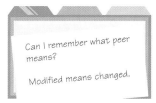

Can I remember what peer means?

Modified means changed.

ACTIVITY 3

Can you think of an occasion when you have modified your verbal or non-verbal behaviour or your appearance to make it more suitable to the people you are with?

Write a short account of it.

Observation Skills to Encourage Communication with Individuals in Different Contexts

We will be exploring the fact that people change their verbal behaviour, non-verbal behaviour and appearance according to the **context** they are in. This may be one to one, in groups of three or more, with their peer group, or with a group including people of different status.

Sometimes behaviour needs to be changed or adjusted because it is not appropriate to the context. Care workers need to be aware of this so that they can take careful notice of their own and other people's behaviour in case it needs to be modified.

Suggestions for such modifications may need to be made by the care worker on the client's behalf. Adults who have **learning difficulties** may be loving and affectionate by nature. It seems a pity to discourage them from showing affection, but it is part of the **normalisation** process to encourage them to behave in an **age-appropriate** manner. Thus we try to teach them that most adults do not kiss the bus driver or cuddle someone to whom they have just been introduced. Encouraging such behaviour sets clients up as objects of ridicule, and is not fair to them.

When we communicate with only one other person, an onlooker can immediately tell our relationship by our non-verbal communication.

unit four

181

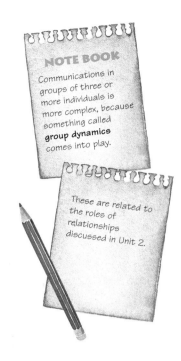

NOTE BOOK

Communications in groups of three or more individuals is more complex, because something called **group dynamics** comes into play.

These are related to the roles of relationships discussed in Unit 2.

This will reflect whether we are with a friend, an acquaintance, a stranger, or someone whom we feel is less or more important than us.

ACTIVITY 4

Work out how you behave differently with a friend, an acquaintance, a stranger, and someone whom you feel is less or more important than yourself, in terms of

- verbal behaviour
- appearance.
- non-verbal behaviour

ACTIVITY 5

1 Imagine you are watching a small group of people

  a at a bus stop   **c** at a meeting.

  b in a cafe

What in their verbal behaviour, non-verbal behaviour and appearance would tell you whether they were friends, work colleagues, employers/employees?

2 Record your conclusions.

Performance Criterion 4

Obstacles to Effective Communication

Many things prevent people from understanding one another. They fall into two categories, environmental obstacles and social and cultural constraints.

Environmental obstacles

The following environmental obstacles prevent effective communication:

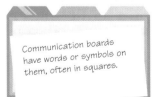

Communication boards have words or symbols on them, often in squares.

People who have difficulty in speaking point to squares to help with communication.

- Distractions – switch the television off and exclude other noises
- Aids not working – spectacles, hearing aid, no communication board, badly fitted false teeth, no pen and pencil to hand
- Impatience – no time allowed for answers or thinking space
- Misinterpreting words and gestures
- Communicating when the client is tired
- Acute infection/illness causing confusion and temporary loss of understanding
- Lack of concentration
- Boredom
- Inappropriate lighting.

Social constraints

It would be nice to think that people felt truly equal to each other. As soon as one feels either superior or inferior to another they begin to have problems in communicating. This may be given away by either their verbal or their non-verbal communication. The messages can be summed up in the expressions

'I'm OK. You're OK.'   (*equal* relationship)

'I'm OK. You're not OK.'

'I'm not OK. You're OK.'   (*inequal* relationship)

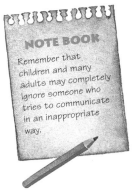

NOTE BOOK

Remember that children and many adults may completely ignore someone who tries to communicate in an inappropriate way.

ACTIVITY 6

For this activity you will work with someone who is **of a different status from yourself**. Before you begin, work out with your colleagues what this means. With this person

1 Discuss the significance of the statement of equality 'I'm OK, you're OK' in the context of communication and interpersonal skills.

2 Work out how being with someone felt to be

   a more important than oneself

   b less important than oneself
   may be an obstacle to effective communication.

3 Record your observations in an appropriate way.

Cultural constraints

The main and most obvious barrier is a language one, but non-verbal communication can cause unintentional offence. In this country we are used to plenty of personal space. We don't stand too close together, we are not particularly demonstrative (that is we don't show emotion), and we may be brought up not to share our feelings. These can all be misinterpreted by people of other cultures, and vice versa. The box on the left shows how one characteristic can be seen as a completely different characteristic by another person/culture.

We need to appreciate the deep differences between cultures so that we do not offend unintentionally and cause others to treat us so warily that true communication becomes impossible.

People's views of people

interested	nosy
polite	cold
enthusiastic	pushy
warm	clinging
affectionate	demanding
articulate	egghead
chatty	noisy

Language

Sometimes we use inappropriate words, give too much information at once, or speak too fast. This is an important consideration when working with clients who themselves have a limited vocabulary, who do not speak English fluently, or who have impaired hearing.

Before being totally accepted into a new group, individuals have to undergo a learning process during which they learn the special words

unit four

and **jargon** of the group. This is more marked when a language other than the native one is involved, such as when people of different nationalities marry and need to communicate with members of one another's extended family. Groups develop jargon, either at work or socially. This excludes those outside the group.

Physical or intellectual constraints

Confused or demented people often respond readily to non-verbal communication and are surprisingly good at picking up messages that the carer had thought had been well hidden like: 'I'm frightened of you'.

Communication impairment

Autism
- no understanding of the meaning of language and social situations
- cannot sympathise with other people's feelings and have few natural social skills
- need to be taught how to behave
- may become excessively anxious when things go wrong
- may not respond warmly or affectionately (which does not mean that we should not respond warmly or affectionately)

Dysarthria
- nerve supply is disrupted making speech slurred e.g. after a stroke
- does not affect understanding, or desire to speak

Dysphasia
- loss of ability to use words properly, e.g. after a stroke nouns are commonly lost, and the client may use words like 'thingummyjig' to fill the gaps.
- sometimes similar sounding words are used wrongly – e.g. 'lock' for 'clock', 'mess' for 'dress'.
- may nod and say 'no' when they mean 'yes'.
- carers need to listen for the meaning and not to the words.

Inappropriate language
- some clients with communication problems pepper their language with recurrent words. These may be quite rude swear words, or phrases like 'I wonder, I wonder, I wonder', with no meaning in the normal sense.

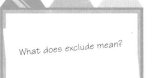
What does exclude mean?

ACTIVITY 7

1 Make a list of jargon words.
2 Record which groups will understand these words, and which groups will be excluded by not understanding them.

Performance Criterion 5

Evaluation of one's own communication skills and suggestions for their improvement

Good communication is an art which can be learned. Some people seem to have been born good communicators, but it is more likely that they have been allowed and enabled to develop good communication skills during their upbringing and schooling.

In order to improve as communicators, we need to be able to work out how good we are already and where improvements need to be made.

There are three stages to this type of evaluation, involving self appraisal, feedback from others, and improvement in methods and techniques.

You will be examining this performance criterion through an activity. You have spent time looking at what helps and what hinders communication. Now you will have a chance to work with what you have learnt.

Note: Remember to be gentle with each other's feelings during the following activities. They are a test of your communication skills. If they become destructive instead of being useful, you will have to re-examine the effectiveness of communications within your group.

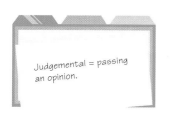

Judgemental = passing an opinion.

ACTIVITY 8

Self-appraisal

Before you go on to find out how you appear to others as a communicator, answer yes or no to the following statements.

A When you talk, do you:

1   maintain eye contact without staring

2   assume other people feel the same as you do about things

3   talk more than you listen

4   use irritating language, such as jargon, slang, or swear words

5   forget that the way you communicate carries messages about the sort of person you are

6   mumble or whisper

7   make sure your listener understands what you are trying to say

8   try to use words that the listener will understand?

To be a good communicator you should answer yes to questions 1, 7, 8 and no to questions 2, 3, 4, 5, 6.

B When you listen do you:

1   jump to conclusions

2   ask for clarification

3   change the subject

4   respond in the right way – for example, being serious when you are being told something important

5   interrupt

6   avoid being judgemental

7   think of your next question, not what is being said

8   react sympathetically instead of feeling threatened

9   pick up little things rather than important ones

10 co-operate rather than compete

11 pretend to understand

12 switch off?

To be a good communicator you should answer yes to questions 2, 4, 6, 8, 10 and no to questions 1, 3, 5, 7, 9, 11, 12.

unit four

ACTIVITY 9

Feedback from others

Select one of the following topics for discussion:

- What I would do if I won the National Lottery.
- What I like about my friends.
- My hobby.
- The time I was most scared.
- Where I would like to live.

Spend five minutes preparing your topic.

Work in groups of three – a speaker, a listener and an observer.

The speaker tells the listener about the chosen topic, while the listener seeks to understand as much as possible at the same time.

Spend five minutes on this.

The observer gives a five minute feedback on what has been seen or heard to help or hinder communication between the two, using the checklist below.

All three in the group will take turns to be the speaker, the listener, and the observer.

Read through the checklist before you start. Record you responses – maybe by video.

CHECKLIST

Speaker	Listener
prepared what was going to be said	didn't take over
clarity of speech	was sympathetic
tone of voice	didn't interrupt
appropriate choice of words	eye contact
eye contact	faced the speaker
logical order of ideas	asked relevant questions
pauses for questions	seemed interested
attitude – friendly	summarised at the end
verbal and non-verbal communication	good body language – didn't fidget
gave the same message	or look bored
	verbal and non-verbal communication gave the same message

Did the speaker behave in a normal way?

Did the listener behave in a normal way for him or her?

Are there ever barriers to effective listening in his or her everyday life?

◀▶ Core skills opportunity:
[NUM 2.1, 2.2., 2.3; IT 2.1, 2.2, 2.3]

1 Present a comparison of how you would spend money won on the National Lottery in the form of a pie chart – e.g. clothes, leisure, holidays, electronic equipment.

2 Collect information about different people's hobbies and present the information in the form of a pie chart and bar chart to stimulate discussion within the group.

3 Collect information about different fears and then categorise before presenting in an appropriate way. Bring in percentages.

4 Collect information about where a group of people would like to live. Express in an appropriate form.

5 Enter these tasks on a spreadsheet and produce the charts and information required using a computer.

ACTIVITY 10

Improvement in techniques

Think about

- open questions
- closed questions
- prompts.

List three examples of each you used/could have used during Activity 2 or during some other recent activity. List three examples of each which other people have used when talking to you recently.

Complete the following table.

How I feel about asking:	
open questions	
closed questions	
probes	
prompts	

1 = not confident   **2** = fairly confident   **3** = confident

ACTIVITY 11

Improvement in methods

Using your findings from Activities 1 and 2, work out how you score in the communication methods shown in the table. Work in pairs.

[Table on the right]

◀▶ **Core skills opportunity [NUM 2.2]**

As members of the group receive a score for each part of the communication section, work out mode, median and mean score.

a for each individual

b for the group.

Discuss the most appropriate form of average to use when choosing a value representative of the group.

Now you know what you need to change.

Methods of verbal and non-verbal communication

Use a scale of **1–5**:   **1** = room for improvements, **2** = not bad, **3** = effective, **4** = very good, **5** = excellent.

Verbal communication methods	1	2	3	4	5
Spoken					
• appropriate level of language					
• appropriate choice of words					
• amount of jargon					
• amount of slang					
• number of swear words					
Written					
• legibility of writing					
• ability to express thoughts					

Non-verbal communication methods	1	2	3	4	5
Tone of voice					
Eye contact					
Facial expression					
Touch/physical contact					
Gestures					
Mime/sign language*					
Body language					
Use of personal space					
Dress/image					
'I'm OK/you're OK' messages					

* delete if not appropriate

unit four

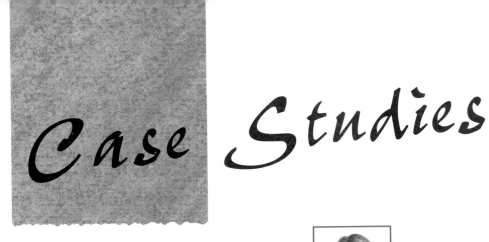

Case Studies

Case study 1   Hill Hall

Ann is rather frightened of Aamon, one of the older children who has a tendency to aggressive behaviour. She likes to keep an eye on him all the time, so she always leaves the door open when toileting him, but this appears to cause him to have outbreaks of temper. Aamon has limited speech, but can communicate with those who have time to persevere.

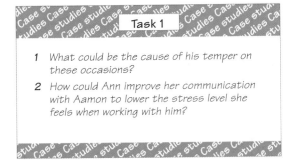

Task 1

1 What could be the cause of his temper on these occasions?
2 How could Ann improve her communication with Aamon to lower the stress level she feels when working with him?

Case study 2   Netherfield Community Care

Mr Dobzanski is a client who is rather fond of Debbie, and she becomes very embarrassed when he starts writing notes to her – 'Debbie means beaty', 'I beleaive in love' etc. She doesn't know how to respond, yet knows she must keep visiting him as part of her duties. She asks Mikhail to help, as she is afraid that Mr Dobzanski will not understand that his attentions are unwelcome, and may assume that she is mocking his poor spelling. He is very sensitive, and Debbie is keen not to offend him.

Mikhail and Debbie need to

1 let Mr Dobzanski know that his behaviour is inappropriate
2 do this without damaging his self-esteem
3 explain to him that they are acknowledging his emotional needs at the same time as Debbie's.

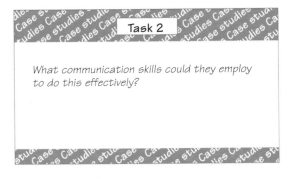

Task 2

What communication skills could they employ to do this effectively?

Case study 3   Down Way School

One day there is a great row in the corridor outside the classroom where Jalwinder is working. A father is threatening loudly to take a baseball bat to his daughter if she doesn't do what the headteacher wants her to do. The head is trying to persuade him to go into her room. All the children are listening with their mouths open, and one of them begins to cry. There are two communication issues here, one between the head and the father, and another between the classroom staff and the children.

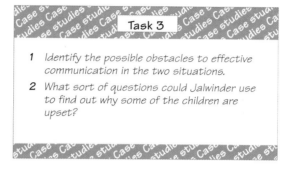

Task 3

1   Identify the possible obstacles to effective communication in the two situations.
2   What sort of questions could Jalwinder use to find out why some of the children are upset?

Case study 4   The Thatched Cottage

It is a big day for Dora. She is going to be assessed for several units of her NVQ by a visiting assessor. Later she tells Mark about it over a cup of tea. She says it was awful. She was nervous, the assessor was very posh and made her feel stupid. She couldn't understand the feedback on her performance. The client they were working with had been really difficult and refused to let Dora put her teeth in. Despite having been successful, Dora is quite upset by the experience. She herself is going to assess Mark for an NVQ element, and promises him that she has learnt a lot about how not to behave when assessing someone.

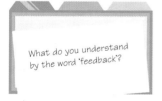

What do you understand by the word 'feedback'?

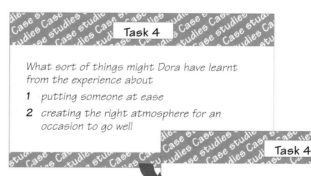

Task 4

What sort of things might Dora have learnt from the experience about

1   putting someone at ease
2   creating the right atmosphere for an occasion to go well

Task 4

3   giving useful feedback after an activity
4   avoiding the barriers to effective communication which arose between herself and the assessor?

unit four case studies

Multiple Choice Questions

1 Which of the following is an example of an open question?

    a *'Did you manage well?'*

    b *'How did you manage after that had happened?'*

    c *'You managed well, did you?'*

    d *'After that, you managed alright, didn't you?'*

2 Self appraisal and feedback are methods of

    a *interpretation*

    b *interaction*

    c *evolution*

    d *evaluation*

3 An unsuitable environment and language misunderstandings are

    a *useful to communication*

    b *obstacles to communication*

    c *methods of communication*

    d *contexts for communication*

4 Which one of the following is a communication skill?

    a *environment*

    b *evaluation*

    c *suitable facial expression*

    d *peer group pressure*

5 Which of the following is an important reason for developing communication skills?

    a *to acknowledge people's beliefs and preferences*

    b *to allow carers to manipulate clients*

    c *for self-appraisal*

    d *to overcome cultural constraints*

6 Verbal communication means

    a *using body language*

    b *listening to people*

    c *speaking to people*

    d *using touch*

Note: These questions are for you to test your knowledge. There is no formal multiple choice test for Unit 4.

Summary of Evidence Opportunities and Their Relationship to Performance Criteria

Activity 1	pc 1	Activities 6 and 7	pc 4	Case study 2	pcs 1, 2 and 3
Activity 2	pc 2	Activities 8, 9, 10 and 11	pc 5	Case study 3	pcs 3 and 4
Activities 3, 4 and 5	pc 3	Case study 1	pcs 1 and 2	Case study 4	pcs 2, 3 and 4

Unit 4 Element 1 Summary of Element Range and Personal Evidence Tracking Record

Element range references *(tick against left-hand column)*	Description of evidence	Pc and range covered	Portfolio reference number
Pc 1 The importance of communication			
self development – intellectual			
– emotional			
– social			
personal beliefs and preferences			
– culture			
– religion			
– politics			
– sexuality			
development of groups			
development of families			
Pc 2 Listening and responding skills			
facial expression			
body language			
eye contact			
sensory contact (touch)			
posture			
minimal prompts			
paraphrasing and summarising			
questioning – open			
– closed			
tone, pitch and pace of communication			
Contexts			
one to one			
groups of three or more			
peer groups			
groups including those of a different status			
Pc 3 Observation skills			
verbal behaviour			
non-verbal behaviour			
appearance			
Contexts as above (pc 2)			

unit four

© *OUP. This page may be photocopied.*

191

Unit 4 Element 1 Summary of Element Range and Personal Evidence Tracking Record

Element range references (tick against left-hand column)	Description of evidence	Pc and range covered	Portfolio reference number
Pc 4 Obstacles to effective communication			
environmental			
social and cultural constraints			
Pc 5 Evaluation			
self appraisal			
feedback from others			
improvements in methods			

Element 4.2

Explore How Inter-Personal Relationships May be Affected by Discriminatory Behaviour

Performance Criteria

pc 1	Provide examples of the different forms which discrimination may take	193
pc 2	Describe behaviours which may indicate discrimination	196
pc 3	Describe how stereotyping individuals and groups can lead to discriminatory behaviour	199
pc 4	Describe the possible effects of discrimination	200
pc 5	Identify the rights which all individuals have under current equality of opportunity legislation	203
	Summary of evidence opportunities and their relationship to the pcs	209
	Summary of element range and personal evidence tracking record	209

Introduction

Discrimination means treating people differently, or making distinctions between them. Discriminatory behaviour affects relationships between individuals and groups in a damaging way.

This element examines the theories and concepts of unfair and unjust discrimination, looking at the forms it may take, behaviour indicating discrimination, the effects of discrimination, and equal opportunities legislation.

Performance Criterion 1

The Different Forms which Discrimination may Take

We will be looking at seven areas which are the common basis for discrimination:

1 age   **4** health status   **6** religion

2 disability   **5** race   **7** sexuality.

3 gender

Age

Individuals are often labelled by their age. Children and young people need protecting during their development, and the following are intended to protect, and are not discriminatory practices.

unit four

- Young people are excluded from places where alcohol is served.

- Young people are not eligible to vote until the age of eighteen.

- It is illegal to sell cigarettes to young people.

- They are excluded from certain forms of employment until a minimum age is reached.

However, speaking in a patronising manner, or ignoring children and young people, is a form of discrimination indicating that they are not being treated as worthwhile individuals.

The reverse happens when older people are treated disrespectfully by others younger than themselves. Some jobs are closed to people in late middle age. In their old age they may be treated like pets or rather large infants.

Disability

Care workers of a generation ago tell how disabled members of families were sometimes kept in a shed at the bottom of the garden with their meals taken down to them. The only work available to them was that which could be undertaken in the shed.

Things have improved since then, but people with physical disabilities are often excluded from jobs in which they could use their intelligence and knowledge despite their handicaps. People with learning disabilities, especially where these are severe, are, sadly, still sometimes treated with little respect.

Consider the options for people who are visually impaired, deaf, or in a wheelchair, and those who have cerebral palsy, autism, and Downs syndrome.

Gender

Men and women are not always treated as equal. This sometimes happens within certain cultural groups where men are seen as being socially superior to women. Ten years ago it was said that women were disadvantaged in education. Currently there is a trend for girls to achieve better GCSE results than boys at 16 years old. The number of women gaining degrees and returning to education as mature students also appears to be increasing proportionately more quickly than the number of men.

In the field of care, most workers are women, and so it is easy to forget that women can be discriminated against in employment. In health care it is men who have to prove themselves as care assistants, midwives, nurses, and health care workers in the same way that women have to in, say, the world of engineering or the fire service.

As single parents, who are most often women, are seen to be bringing children up successfully, young men may begin to feel inadequate. They may lack male role models, especially if they attend a school with mainly female teachers.

Traditionally women in our society remain the main carers. They are expected to look after elderly relatives, maybe sacrificing their own chance of marriage to do so. It is far less common for men to take on this role.

Health status

The table on the left shows examples of groups which may be discriminated against.

Race

Race, culture and ethnic origin are closely linked. **Race** is to do with people's physical characteristics, for example the colour of their skin and eyes, the shape of their faces, or hair characteristics.

Ethnicity, ethnic origin and **culture** determine which clothes people wear, their behaviour with each other, what they eat, and the language they use. An **ethnic minority** is a cultural group not widely represented in the area in which its people live.

Religion

Religion crosses race and cultural boundaries. The main world religions are Buddhism, Christianity, Hinduism and Islam (practised by Muslims). Sadly, many of the worst wars are fought in the name of religion, even between sects of the same religion.

In the area of mental health
- people with schizophrenia
- depression
- behavioural problems

In the area of physical health
- people with epilepsy
- people who are Aids/HIV positive
- people who have an ileostomy / colostomy

In a range of categories
- people who are homeless
- drug abusers
- people with alcohol-related problems
- those who have been in prison
- travelling families

Groups which may experience discrimination

Ileostomy/colostomy = an artificial opening into the bowel fitted with a disposable bag to collect waste matter.

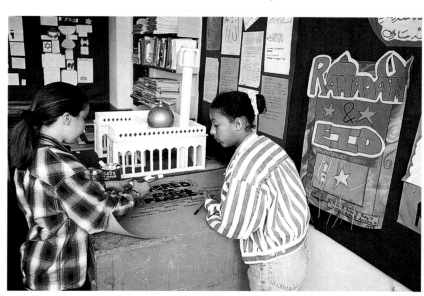

Countries with a rich and diverse history, such as the United Kingdom and the USA, have representatives of very many races and cultures living together. They are said to be **multi-racial** and **multi-cultural** societies.

It is discriminatory not to allow a person or group to practise their cultural beliefs in a way appropriate to them, or not to provide food acceptable to them when they are in a care-setting.

unit four

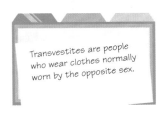

Transvestites are people who wear clothes normally worn by the opposite sex.

Sexuality

Examples of groups who may be discriminated against in our society include homosexual men, lesbians, and transvestites.

People's sexuality is a private matter. It may be complicated and unusual, and there is no reason why it should be made public. It is only when it breaks the law that it needs to be discussed with other people.

Carers are in a privileged position in that they often hear clients' most personal secrets. They are also vulnerable, as they may discover something which they personally find distasteful. The boundaries of confidentiality are explored in Element 4.3.

Performance Criterion 2

Direct
abusive language
ignoring the individual
obvious offensive behaviour
offensive jokes
not touching

Indirect
tone of voice
withholding support
body language
exclusion from advice
avoidance

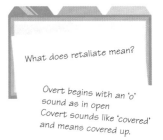

What does retaliate mean?

Overt begins with an 'o' sound as in open
Covert sounds like 'covered' and means covered up.

Behaviours which may Indicate Discrimination

Discrimination may be **direct** or **indirect**.

Direct discriminatory behaviour

Abusive language

People whose appearance makes them stand out may be subjected to abusive language, Racial groups, people with obvious disabilities and those who dress differently from the majority are particularly likely to suffer in this way.

Verbal abuse is often a result of extreme stereotyping. It is not necessarily caused by hatred; it may show that the person being abused is considered to be of inferior status and seen to be lacking the power to retaliate. Abusive language is a form of emotional abuse. It is not always obvious, but whispers can be very sinister. Mockery, put-downs and name-calling are all examples of abusive language.

Obvious offensive behaviour

The word used for this is **overt**, which means it can be seen. The opposite is **covert** which means it is hidden. Overt offensive behaviour ranges from pushing or spitting to physical harm, such as attacks with an anti-racial motive or against homosexuals.

Children and old people are sometimes treated roughly. Men and women are sometimes subjected to offensive behaviour which amounts to sexual harassment.

Sexual abuse is an extreme form of overt offensive behaviour. It can occur for discriminatory reasons, to enforce power, to humiliate, or for gratification with someone who cannot protect themselves and who is regarded therefore as being inferior.

Not touching

Lepers used to ring a bell to warn people they were coming so that they could be avoided. If today we choose to withhold touch from someone, we are denying them their social acceptability.

Some groups of people who may be avoided because of prejudice are

- those who are HIV positive
- those who have skin complaints
- those of a different race or culture
- elderly people
- people who are incontinent
- people who are deformed or ugly.

Some cultures by tradition have a caste system, in which society is divided according to rank and importance. The lowest caste of some cultures that used to be in existence in India was that of the Untouchables, people considered too inferior even to be near.

Racist or sexist jokes

It is often those who feel most threatened who feel the need to make racist or sexist jokes. Although people who object to them may be accused of lacking a sense of humour, they are right to, as these jokes reinforce race or sex stereotypes in a harmful way.

Ignoring

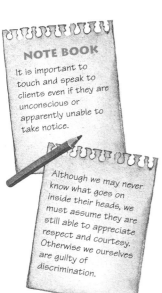

Prejudice comes from 'pre-judge', and means making up your mind beforehand.

NOTE BOOK

It is important to touch and speak to clients even if they are unconscious or apparently unable to take notice.

Although we may never know what goes on inside their heads, we must assume they are still able to appreciate respect and courtesy. Otherwise we ourselves are guilty of discrimination.

NOTE BOOK

People with learning difficulties or mental health problems often relate more to tone of voice than to the words which are spoken.

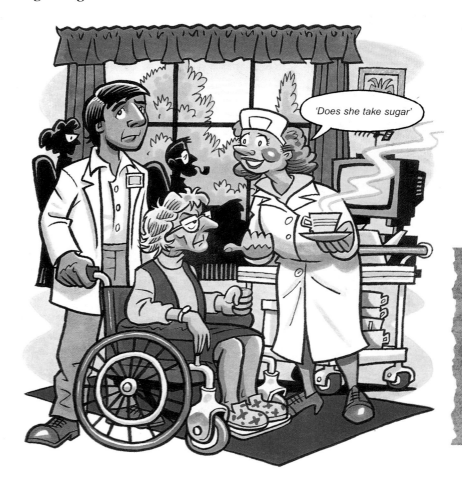

'Does she take sugar'

unit four

197

We are offended if a shop assistant carries on a private conversation while we wait to be served. It makes us feel small. Likewise, clients feel excluded if two carers chat over their heads without including them in their conversation.

Indirect discriminatory behaviour

Tone of voice

It can be discriminatory to sound patronising, sneering, disapproving, suggestive, angry, or sarcastic. We can express all these feelings not by our choice of words but by the way in which they are spoken. Likewise, when you hear a foreign language it is easy to guess the mood of the conversation by the tone of voice used by the speakers.

Body language

If a person is not to feel rejected, our body language needs to make them feel accepted. The table on the left looks at examples of rejecting and accepting body language.

Avoidance

People who have had a dreadful personal misfortune, such as death of a loved one or bad news of severe illness, report that their friends sometimes cross the road to avoid speaking to them. This is very hurtful. When it is done from discriminatory motives it is extremely insulting.

Exclusion from advice

Recently a black woman, who was overweight to a degree which was life-threatening, stated that she was offered no health care advice to encourage her to lose weight. It was not until she found a doctor from her own ethnic background that she received information which was realistic and understandable.

A small group of elderly people in the UK has Aids. They complain that no support is appropriate for them; all Aids literature is aimed at young people.

When someone speaks English fairly fluently, but not as their first language, it may not be obvious if they do not understand everything which is said. Advice may be denied to people because they cannot read, cannot read English, or have difficulty understanding if the information is not presented in a pictorial or simple style.

Young adults with learning disabilities need access to health promotion advice and support with regard to their sexuality. To assume that they don't is to deny them their rights.

How our body language speaks

Ways to reject

avoiding eye contact
arms folded
standing at a distance
leaning over a person
not smiling
hands on hips

Ways to accept

making eye contact
relaxing the hands and shoulders
not standing too far away
sitting down next to someone in a wheelchair or in a bed
smiling

An example of direct discrimination

An Asian person is not offered a job because he or she is Asian.

An example of indirect discrimination

An employer devises a test which is culturally biased so that an Asian candidate is likely to fail.

Performance Criterion 3

How Stereotyping Individuals and Groups can Lead to Discriminatory Behaviour

When we **stereotype** a person or a group we stop seeing people as individuals and mass them together under a single label which robs them of personality. Using stereotypes is a lazy way of thinking – it saves the trouble of finding out more about people.

Stereotyping begins with making assumptions, which may be based on our first impressions:

- use of language
- accent
- area they live in
- education
- clothes
- car/house ownership
- occupation.

All these and more affect the way we first feel about people. If we do not get to know them better they may remain fixed in our minds as stereotypes.

Advertisements, magazines and television all feed stereotypes. Drama often portrays people as shallow images with no past or future. Advertisements depict ideal situations with no problems or personal hardships. Magazines show rose-tinted, unattainable situations, which the average person cannot hope to achieve.

ACTIVITY 1

1 Find an advertisement showing a stereotyped individual, group or situation.

2 Describe it as the advertiser wishes you to see it.

3 Imagine what might be the reality behind the stereotype.

4 Think of the disadvantages which might follow the portrayal of an ideal rather than a real image as far as the reader is concerned.

5 Draw some speech bubbles coming out of the mouths of those in the picture contradicting the image presented in the illustration.

6 Use the activity to produce a page suitable for inclusion in a student leaflet designed to raise awareness of discriminatory behaviour. Use a computer if you wish.

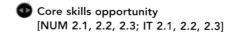 **Core skills opportunity**
[NUM 2.1, 2.2, 2.3; IT 2.1, 2.2, 2.3]

Conduct a survey among your colleagues to see how many different types of stereotype they have identified. Choosing a cross-section of about 30 people you know, see how many could fit into each of the stereotypes you have identified. Present your information in the form of a suitable chart, and maybe draw conclusions from the graphical display by expressing these opinions in the form of probability.

When we see people as 'cardboard cut-outs' with no blood in their veins, feelings in their minds or personal histories, dreams or disappointments, we are stereotyping them. By denying them an existence as individuals we cease to have sympathy for them and the seeds of discrimination are sown.

unit four

Performance Criterion 4

The Possible Effects of Discrimination

When people experience discrimination, the results are negative and harmful. The effects of this can be short term or long term in which case they can be much more serious.

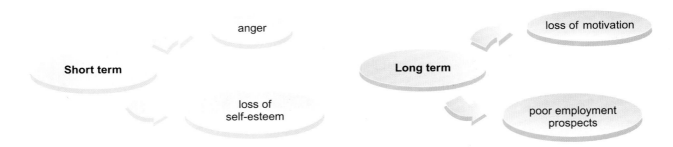

Short term

Anger

Anger can act as a positive or negative force. Some anger is directed at self-improvement, while more usually it is used destructively to destroy material things – property, gardens, cars – or abstract things – relationships, self-image, opportunities.

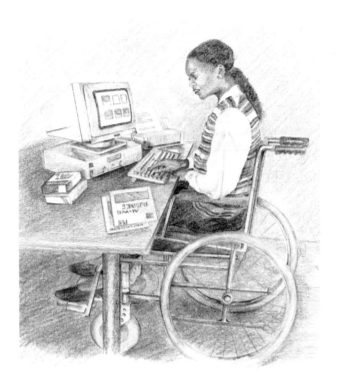

Determined anger (assertive behaviour)
'I'll show them what I'm capable of!

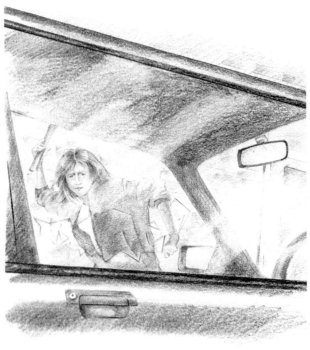

Destructive anger (aggressive behaviour)
'I'll show them.'

Loss of self-esteem (self-worth)

Everybody can understand loss of self-esteem, so it is within all of us to be able to sympathise with how people experiencing discrimination must feel for much of the time. We may all experience it occasionally. For many it is a permanent state.

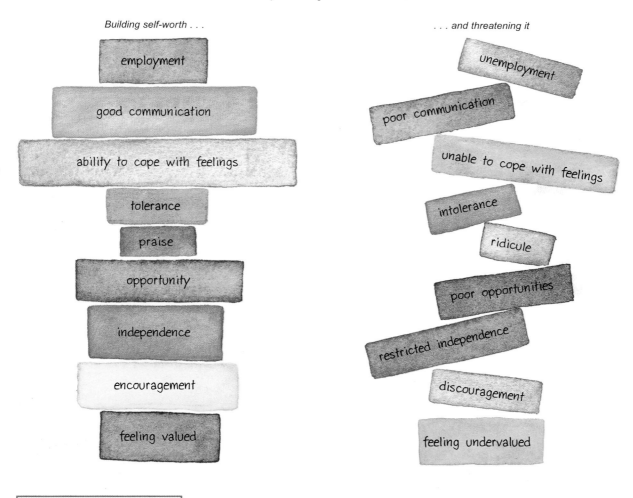

Building self-worth . . .

- employment
- good communication
- ability to cope with feelings
- tolerance
- praise
- opportunity
- independence
- encouragement
- feeling valued

. . . and threatening it

- unemployment
- poor communication
- unable to cope with feelings
- intolerance
- ridicule
- poor opportunities
- restricted independence
- discouragement
- feeling undervalued

ACTIVITY 2

1 Look back at Element 2.1 where individual's development and self-concepts were explored.

2 Discuss how discrimination will affect people's self-concept when they are unable to find meaningful employment because of **three** of the following bases of discrimination:

- age/youth
- gender
- race
- health status.
- disability

3 Draw up a survey by asking people which form of discrimination they regard as being the reason for employers not offering people jobs. Present the information in graphical form and draw conclusions from the graph in numerical form – e.g. mean, mode, probability. **[NUM 2.1, 2.3]**

unit four

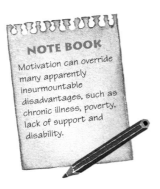

NOTE BOOK

Motivation can override many apparently insurmountable disadvantages, such as chronic illness, poverty, lack of support and disability.

Long term

Detrimental employment prospects

Stereotyped attitudes are self-confirming. If poorly paid jobs which most of society does not want to do are the only ones in which people of certain groups manage to gain employment, then it is easy to form the opinion that those are the only jobs they are able to do.

Ultimately such employees may become resigned to thinking they are capable of nothing better, when in reality they may have other talents worthy of being developed if the opportunity arose.

Lack of motivation

Motivation is the inner force which drives us to do things. The diagram below illustrates some of the many sources of motivation.

Driving Force

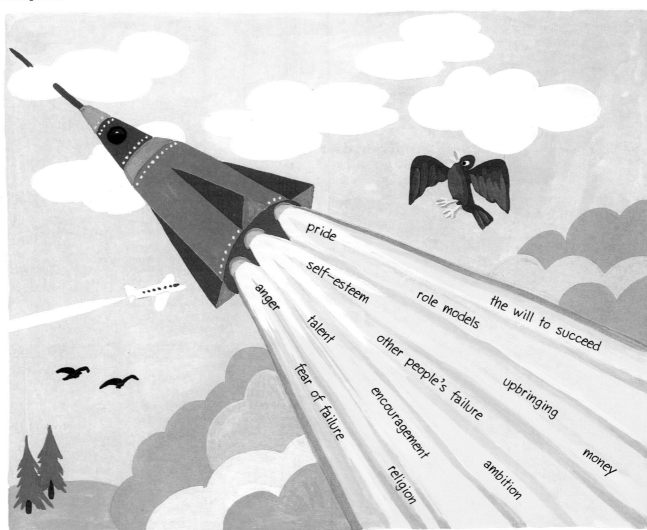

ACTIVITY 3

1 Using the figure below, work out whether these motivational forces may work for (use a tick '✓') or against (use a cross '✗') groups who are discriminated against.

⬤ **Core skills opportunity**
[NUM 2.1, 2.2, 2.3; IT 2.1, 2.2, 2.3]

Taking into consideration the different sources of motivation, conduct a survey to find out if motivation sources might be linked to different types of discrimination. Express your conclusion either in graphical form or statistical analysis. Use a computer, save on disk and print.

2 You will find the answers are not straightforward. Discuss why this should be so.

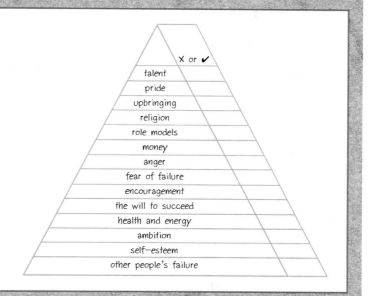

Performance Criterion 5

Individual's Rights Under Current Equality of Opportunity Legislation

Laws have been drawn up to protect citizens from discrimination.

These are:

		relating to
1	Sex Discrimination Acts 1975 and 1986	*gender*
2	Race Relations Act 1976	*race*
3	The Chronically Sick and Disabled Persons Act 1970 and 1986	*disability*
4	Equal Pay Act 1970/1988	*pay*
5	Fair Employment Act (NI) 1989	*employment*

Sex Discrimination Acts 1975 and 1986

These Acts were designed to prevent discrimination on the grounds of gender. They make it illegal to discriminate in

- employment
- access to goods and services
- education
- other areas of life

unit four

by

- treating one gender less favourably
- attaching conditions to jobs which make them impossible for some candidates to get interviews
- sexual harassment or victimisation – this applies to men as well as women
- setting age limits to exclude those who might be involved in child care
- dismissing women who become pregnant.

The **Equal Opportunities Commission** monitors and advises people who feel they have been victims of discrimination on the grounds of their gender.

Its role is

- to work towards the elimination of discrimination on the basis of gender
- to promote equality between men and women
- to review the Sex Discrimination and Equal Pay Acts
- to support research related to equal opportunities for men and women.

The Race Relations Act 1976

This act makes it illegal to encourage racial hatred or to discriminate on the grounds of

- race
- colour
- ethnic origin
- nationality.

It covers the provision of goods, facilities and services, employment, housing and advertising. The Race Relations Act is monitored by the **Commission for Racial Equality**, which relies on central and local government, the police, the Director for Public Prosecutions and other bodies to enforce the law.

The Chronically Sick Act 1975, The Disabled Persons Act 1986

Under these Acts social services departments are required to assess the needs of people with disabilities who live in their area. Needs assessed are

practical needs

- personal care needs
- help in the home and with meals

NOTE BOOK

It is important not to get carried away by your convictions – not all girls want to be mechanics, nor do all boys want to work in a creche.

The challenge is to give people the chance to consider a range of opportunities and let them decide for themselves.

NOTE BOOK

Racial discrimination can be discouraged by prosecution, persuasion and education. However, it is difficult to enforce laws when discrimination is hidden.

It is easier to prosecute cases of racial discrimination than to change deeply embedded attitudes in society.

transport needs

- car adaptations

- vehicle able to carry a wheelchair

- transport which can be got into and out of easily

leisure and communication needs

- television

- telephone

- talking books

designers and owners of new buildings must consider the access needs

- for people with disabilities, such as, ramps and lifts, toilet adaptations, etc. Since the 1981 Disabled Persons Act, planning permission has to give consideration to access for people with disabilities. Access Officers are sometimes employed by local authorities to manage these regulations.

The second Act (1986) has not yet been fully implemented and at present (1995) there is pressure to put this right. It covers:

- the main carer's ability to provide care

- provision of information of services available across statutory, voluntary, and private sectors

- consultation with organisations of people with disabilities before an individual is appointed to represent them on council committees.

The Equal Pay Act 1970/1988 (amended)

This Act is concerned with all aspects of ensuring equal pay for equal work for all.

Once a man in a job would earn more than a woman in the same job. This was the case in teaching as well as the armed forces and many other occupations. Now this is illegal, as it is for pay to be linked to able-bodied status, culture, race or religion.

The Equal Opportunities Commission monitors and advises on all aspects of this Act as well as the Sex Discrimination Act.

Fair Employment Act (NI) 1989

This Act, which concerns only Northern Ireland, covers the same issues as the Act previously discussed.

ACTIVITY 4

◀▶ **Extension opportunity**
The **Children Act 1989** and the **Diability Access Act 1995** affect many aspects of care. Find out more about them and summarise some of their main effects.

unit four

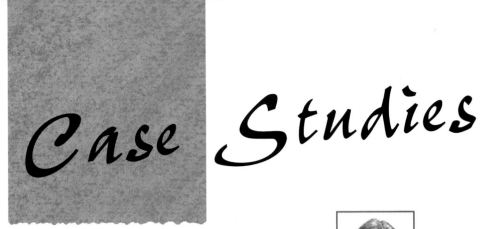

Case Studies

Case study 1   Down Way School
(continued from Element 4.1)

Jalwinder goes out to see if she can help and the father calls her 'a scrawny little Paki'. Jalwinder loses her temper, which is rare for her, and shouts back that the parent is discriminating against her. Later in the playground she overhears the children repeating 'scrawny little Paki' as the chorus to a skipping game.

Task 1

1 How could the staff at the school explain the meaning of discrimination to the children?

2 Would children find it easier to understand the short or the long term effects of discrimination?

Task 2

1 What forms of discrimination are being exhibited?

2 How is the discrimination being demonstrated?

Task 2

3 Is Gertrude being discriminatory, stereotyping, or neither?

4 Discuss your answers in a group.

Case study 2   The Thatched Cottage

Mark takes some of the residents to the nearby pub every Thursday for a drink before lunch, pushing Bill in his wheelchair. He began the habit to celebrate his 18th birthday and has continued with it ever since. He gets annoyed with one of the bar staff who speaks to him instead of Bill when the drinks are being ordered, and with a woman who complains loudly about the residents lowering the tone of the establishment. Luckily the pub manager is on Mark's side, and has a word with the bar person, and makes it clear to the woman that The Thatched Cottage residents are always welcome. Gertrude finds this encouraging, and, after downing a glass of stout, launches into a graphic account of the joys of being bathed by Mark.

Case study 3   Hill Hall

Outside the walls of Hill Hall there is much opportunity for discrimination. Molly's race and colour, and the children's learning difficulties and sometimes bizarre behaviour make them easy targets for discriminatory behaviour. Molly likes to take some of the children to a local hypermarket to help them to see everyday life. One day she is jostled by a shopper who tells her to get her 'great dirty hands off the bread'. One of the children catches Molly's distress and begins to throw buns at the shopper. The manager is called, and threatens the shopper with legal action. The shopper retaliates with a threat because there are no toilet adaptations for disabled people (which is irrelevant, but true).

Task 3

1 Which Acts could the manager and the shopper be penalised under?

2 If the hypermarket manager sacked a staff member because she was pregnant, or paid paperboys more than papergirls, which other Acts would be broken?

Case study 4   Netherfield Community Care

There is a significant degree of unemployment in the town. The prison service has a help line for ex-offenders, and anyone needing a sympathetic ear can ring at any time of day or night. It becomes obvious that, after coming out of prison, the young men in particular are not being offered job interviews. The local community decides to address this matter.

Task 4

1 What legislation is there in your area to help this group of people to secure jobs?

2 What are the likely effects of discrimination of this sort on the young men of Netherfield, which makes it desirable to act on their behalf before too much time passes?

Task 4

3 What might be the stereotyping which leads to discrimination against ex-offenders applying for jobs?

✦ Extension opportunity

Look in the media for evidence of discrimination leading to detrimental job prospects. Use the seven different forms of discrimination. Remember that 'the media' includes television, radio and written material. Select an appropriate format for your findings. Employ Core Skills imaginatively.

unit four case studies

Multiple Choice Questions

1 Calling someone a white fascist is an example of discriminatory behaviour which is

    a *covert*

    b *indirect*

    c *overt*

    d *sexist*

2 Which of the following is an example of the basis of discrimination?

    a *anger*

    b *age*

    c *motivation*

    d *stereotype*

3 Which of the following might be a long-term effect of discrimination?

    a *lack of motivation*

    b *abusive language*

    c *stereotyping*

    d *indirect behaviour*

4 Which action would best be described as *indirect* discriminatory behaviour?

    a *not touching someone believed to be HIV positive*

    b *using abusive language to a confused client*

    c *ignoring a person in a wheelchair*

    d *using a tone of voice which ridicules a Chinese woman*

5 Stereotyping means

    a *thinking that all people in a group are the same*

    b *behaving badly towards people with disabilities*

    c *avoiding people who have a different religion*

    d *telling racist jokes*

6 Which of the following Acts makes it compulsory for architects to design public buildings with ramps for access?

    a *the Race Relations Act*

    b *the Sex Discrimination Act*

    c *the Equal Pay Act*

    d *the Disabled Persons Act*

Note: These questions are for you to test your knowledge. There is no formal multiple choice test for Unit 4.

Summary of Evidence Opportunities and Their Relationship to Performance Criteria

Activity 1	pc 3	**Case study 1**	pcs all	**Case study 4**	pcs 3, 4 and 5
Activity 2	pc 4	**Case study 2**	pcs 1, 2 and 3		
Activity 3	pc 4	**Case study 3**	pc 5		

Unit 4 Element 2 Summary of Element Range and Personal Evidence Tracking Record

Element range references (*tick against left-hand column*)	Description of evidence	Pc and range covered	Portfolio reference number
Pc 1 Bases of discrimination			
age			
disability			
gender			
health status			
race			
religion			
sexuality			
Pc 2 Discriminatory behaviours			
direct			
indirect			
Pc 3 Stereotyping			
Pc 4 Effects of discrimination			
short-term			
– anger			
– loss of self-esteem			
long-term			
– detrimental employment prospects			
– lack of motivation			
Pc 5 Equal opportunities legislation			
relating to – gender			
– race			
– disability			
– pay			
– employment			

unit four

© OUP. This page may be photocopied.

Element 4.3

Investigate Aspects of Working with Clients in Health and Social Care

Performance Criteria		
pc 1	Describe how the caring relationship may differ in nature from other forms of relationship	210
pc 2	Explain ways in which clients may respond to being in receipt of care	215
pc 3	Describe how different types of support may affect inter-personal relationships between clients and carers	218
pc 4	Describe the role of effective interaction in caring relationships	221
pc 5	Explain why confidentiality is of critical importance in health and social care settings	224
pc 6	Explain the ethical issues which individuals may face in relation to maintaining confidentiality	226
	Summary of evidence opportunities and their relationship to the pcs	231
	Summary of element range and personal evidence tracking record	231

Introduction

The final element in Unit 4 brings together the element on communication skills with that on discriminatory behaviour, and expands them to examine the interpersonal relationships formed in the field of health and social care.

Performance Criterion 1

How the Caring Relationship May Differ in Nature From Other Forms of Relationship

The caring relationship is unique in the world of employment as one person, **the carer**, and another, **the client**, enter into a professional partnership that appears to be unequal. The carer can be seen as being independent, with the client dependent. The carer appears to have power, while the client may appear to be helpless.

We examine the undercurrents below these assumptions to find what is desirable about the carer/client relationship and what is not. Dependence of clients and carers, the extent to which clients can be self-managing, the perceived equality of the relationship, perceived power within the relationship, and perceived knowledge and understanding about the situation are considered in turn.

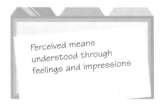

Perceived means understood through feelings and impressions

Dependence of clients and carers

All clients appear to be dependent on their carers, whether the caring is informal or professional.

ACTIVITY 1

carer	client
parent	baby
baby-sitter	elderly parent
adult child	parishioner
clergyman	child
nurse	client at home
care assistant	baby
dentist	resident
health care worker	patient
classroom assistant	pupil
nanny	family in the community
teacher	school child
social worker	patient

1 Decide

   a which client might be linked with which carer

   b which is an informal relationship and which is a professional one

   c which pairs of client and carer might be connected with each of the four case study contexts.

2 Work out which of the carers listed offer support which is a social; b financial; c physical; d emotional; e giving information.

   Some carers may fall into more than one category. Design a graph or table to show your conclusions. **[NUM 2.1, 2.3]**

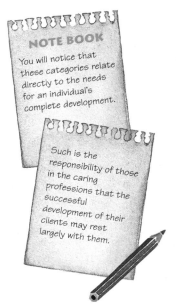

NOTE BOOK

You will notice that these categories relate directly to the needs for an individual's complete development.

Such is the responsibility of those in the caring professions that the successful development of their clients may rest largely with them.

Dependence is the opposite of independence, and means **relying on someone**. It has undertones of being inferior, which is why it must be managed tactfully. In caring the aim is to allow clients to be as independent as they can be within the limitations of their age, physical or mental condition, or emotional state.

Dependence can be **physical, intellectual, emotional**, or **financial**, or a combination of them.

Types of dependence

Physical	- means that there is reliance for food, hygiene, mobility, clothing, etc.
Emotional	- means that support, encouragement and praise must constantly reinforce a client's self-esteem.
Intellectual	- means stimulus needs to be provided to allow a person to develop fully.
Financial	- means that a client cannot make ends meet without monetary help.

It is in the nature of relationships that the personalities of those concerned become intertwined. Some carers become dependent on their clients, for example

- as children grow older their mothers may find it hard to let them become fully independent

unit four

ACTIVITY 2

Return to the list of client/carers in Activity 1. Work out whether the client is dependent physically, emotionally or financially on the carer, or what combination of the three applies. The table on p. 211 will help you do this.

- some carers go off duty late because they feel indispensable to those in their care
- a client may take the place of a child to a childless carer
- a carer may be reluctant to leave a group of clients for a promotion or career move as they feel safe with the clients they know and like
- adult children with dependent parents may choose not to lead an independent life as they build up an existence centred round the parent they look after.

It is unkind to treat clients like babies because it robs them of dignity. It often stems from a carer's urge to feel wanted rather than an actual need of the client.

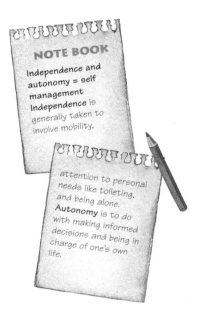

NOTE BOOK

Independence and autonomy = self management
Independence is generally taken to involve mobility,

attention to personal needs like toileting, and being alone.
Autonomy is to do with making informed decisions and being in charge of one's own life.

The extent to which clients can be self-managing

All carers must aim to help clients to be as independent and as autonomous as possible.

ACTIVITY 3

1 Think about
   a a bedridden patient
   b a small child
   c a person in a wheelchair
   d a person suffering from schizophrenia
   e a family on a very low income.
   List the factors affecting their independence and autonomy.
2 Work out which clients might be connected with each case study establishment.

You will find that there are similarities and differences between the clients in Activity 3, affecting how self-managing they can be. The carer's aim is to make sure that every client is as independent and autonomous as possible within their personal abilities.

Self-management has an element of risk, which some carers find frightening. All independence involves some risk.

The perceived equality of the relationship

Element 4.1 looks briefly at the 'I'm OK, you're OK' situation in which mutual respect is emphasised. As soon as client and carer lose sight of this, the relationship becomes unbalanced in ways which will be explored in pc 2 of this element.

Client and carer need to work together in partnership towards making the client as self-managing as possible. It cannot be achieved if one of the two loses sight of this aim. The balance is lost if:

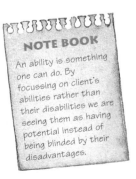

NOTE BOOK

An ability is something one can do. By focussing on client's abilities rather than their disabilities we are seeing them as having potential instead of being blinded by their disadvantages.

- the carer becomes patronising

- the client loses motivation

- the carer allows the client to become dependent

- the client is treated like a pet

- communication breaks down

- the client is encouraged to behave in a way inappropriate for his/her age

One of the benefits of care in the community is that carers can meet clients in their homes, where they can be seen as individuals with families and belongings and a private life of their own.

Perceived power within the relationship

The carer's role has an element of power in it. Think about the power in the following roles: parent, doctor, teacher, prison officer, health visitor, nurse, policeman.

ACTIVITY 4

1 Discuss how the following attributes contribute to feelings of power:

- health
- personality
- mobility
- money
- vocabulary
- size
- education
- freedom

2 Now turn the situation upside down. Consider the power which could be wielded by the following types of client:

- toddler
- hospital patient
- older person
- student
- prisoner
- family in the community

3 What behaviour might they show to demonstrate their power?

4 Record you conclusions imaginatively, using Core Skills where you can.

What is a malpractice?

All carers and their clients are first and foremost individuals with personalities, and this is what decides whether they choose to display their power and to what extent.

When someone uses power, other people feel disadvantaged and inferior. It is a tool with which to manipulate, whether used by a client or a carer.

In a client/carer relationship the carer is the stronger, and should be able to suppress any desire to make the client feel small. Any other behaviour is unprofessional and unbecoming, leading to malpractices such as physical and emotional abuse of clients.

unit four

ACTIVITY 5

1 Return to Activity 4 and the list of attributes contributing to power.

2 Work out ways in which they could be used positively on clients' behalf.

3 Adjust your records to include your findings.

Instances of mis-use of power include the use of sarcasm, verbal abuse, rough handling, bullying, teasing, sexual abuse, withholding food, and withholding approval. However power can be used positively, from advocacy on clients' behalf to influencing local groups to provide facilities.

Perceived knowledge and understanding of the situation

You will by now realise the need for effective communication between clients and their carers. If clients are to understand what is going on around them, it must be explained to them in an appropriate way.

Many of the procedures carried out by carers seem quite bizarre if the reason behind them is not understood. This is why they need explaining clearly and carefully beforehand to clients in a way they can understand. It reinforces understanding if relatives and friends also understand procedures, possible effects of treatment, and social constraints.

ACTIVITY 6

Imagine the following happening to you:
1 Having a needle stuck in your thigh.
2 Having all your clothes taken off.
3 Your hair falling out.
4 Door handles being out of your reach.
5 Total loss of income.
6 Having to be in bed by 7.30 pm.
7 Falling over all the time.
8 Not being allowed to eat or drink.
9 Suddenly not seeing a loved one ever again.
10 Having to take tablets 3 times a day when you feel perfectly well.

Now match the following reasons for these situations and discuss them.
a A child's need for rest.
b Chemotherapy.
c A fatal road accident.
d Awaiting anaesthetic.
e Medication for drug-controlled complaint.
f Bath time.
g Stroke.
h Unsafe to go out alone.
i Antibiotic injection.
j Redundancy

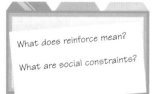

What does reinforce mean?

What are social constraints?

The carer is similarly disadvantaged if clients do not or cannot share background information, such as current medication, domestic difficulties, and financial problems. Remember that information is usually withheld by clients because of embarrassment, not knowing it is relevant, or lack of forethought, rather than an intentional wish to be unco-operative.

Information may be withheld by the carer for the same reason. This may be avoided by good team-building, effective communication between staff, and training.

Performance Criterion 2

Ways in Which Clients May Respond to Being in Receipt of Care

Some people see the good side of receiving care – **positive responses** – while others find it difficult to accept – **negative responses**. Here we look at the reasons which may underlie the two attitudes.

Positive responses

Positive responses to receiving care might be feeling relaxed, feeling relieved, reduced stress, and reduced worry about coping.

Feeling relaxed

Relaxed clients take everything in their stride. This may be because they understand and are supportive of the care or treatment they are receiving, because of their personality, or because their level of understanding is reduced to a point that they accept whatever turns up in life.

Feeling relieved

When people have found a situation or complaint tiresome or worrying, they feel that a weight has been taken off their shoulders when it is being resolved or addressed. For example a definite diagnosis of an illness may be a relief after a lengthy series of tests.

Reduced stress

There is a saying that a sick individual means a sick family, meaning that everyone involved with someone with problems is affected to some degree. When a client begins to receive attention, any lowering of stress is usually shared by the family, meaning that tension in the client's relationships are eased, which is always beneficial.

Reduced worry about coping

We all become anxious about our ability to cope at one time or another. When people are ill or have social problems, they are frequently relieved when someone else begins to take over some responsibility, and they can see that their difficulties are acknowledged and shared.

Negative responses

Negative responses to being in care include stress or distress, withdrawal, difficulty in expressing feelings, and aggression or abuse.

Stress or distress

Some people are unwilling to accept that they or their loved ones need help or care. They find it difficult to come to terms with, and become increasingly anxious and worried.

Distress is a feeling of pain, grief and calamity deeper than stress, and more immediate. It may be felt, for instance, when someone finds out

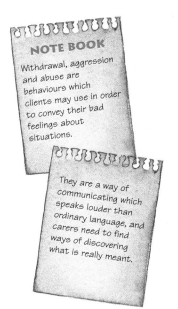

NOTE BOOK

Withdrawal, aggression and abuse are behaviours which clients may use in order to convey their bad feelings about situations.

They are a way of communicating which speaks louder than ordinary language, and carers need to find ways of discovering what is really meant.

unit four

ACTIVITY 7

1 Think of other situations which can cause distress.

2 Can you draw any parallels between them and bereavement?

◀▶ **Core skills opportunity [NUM 2.1, 2.2, 2.3; IT 2.1, 2.2, 2.3]**

- Work out a way of estimating people's responses to distress, such as a scale of 1-10.

- Apply your chosen method to the possible responses to the situations you have identified above.

- Illustrate using graphs and diagrams.

- Use a computer to present your findings, save on disk and print.

they have an incurable illness, a relationship is being ended, an operation is needed, or a prison sentence has been imposed.

Distress levels, like stress levels, are personal, and vary according to the individual. Some people are better able to cope with shocks than others. Remember that troubles do not always come singly. A person who is already ill may also have bad news about the family – one misfortune does not exempt people from others. Degrees of stress and distress are both normal in everyday life experiences. Many of the situations causing distress are forms of bereavement (See also Unit 2, Element 2.1, pc 3). The bereavement may take the form of

- a severe illness, which deprives us of health

- a severed friendship, which deprives us of a relationship

- an operation, which deprives us of part of our body

- a prison sentence, which deprives us of freedom.

A period of adjustment is needed, just as it is after a death. This is why distress is seldom a permanent emotion.

Withdrawal

Withdrawal may show itself in all or some of the following ways:

- indifference to surroundings

- aloof or detached attitudes

- keeping away from other people

- non-communicative body language

- short, brief answers to questions

- not readily talking to others

- refusing to speak

- substituting fantasy for the real world.

If a carer becomes responsible for a client showing these tendencies, they should first make sure that they are not symptoms of their illness. If the symptoms develop in an otherwise outward-going, communicative person, then warning bells need to sound and the care team must investigate.

Difficulty in expressing feelings

Negative responses to needing care may only be shown by clients' behaviour. They are unlikely to say 'I have an increased stress level' or 'I feel distressed' because most human beings find it hard to express their emotions in such a straightforward way. We are too complicated for that.

In addition, clients are frequently disadvantaged by being unable to understand what is going on, not having the right vocabulary to express their fears, or being brought up to hide their true feelings.

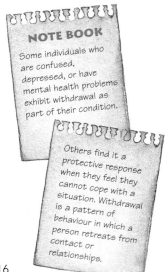

NOTE BOOK

Some individuals who are confused, depressed, or have mental health problems exhibit withdrawal as part of their condition.

Others find it a protective response when they feel they cannot cope with a situation. Withdrawal is a pattern of behaviour in which a person retreats from contact or relationships.

The complexities of the caring relationship as described in pc 1 makes this worse.

Aggression or abuse

Aggression is a normal human emotion. Like withdrawal, aggression is frequently a problem of mental illness, and may stem from hallucinations or misinterpretation of surroundings. It may also be an individual's only known way of gaining attention or reward, because he/she has not learnt how to express anger or aggressive energy in a more acceptable way. On the other hand a formerly polite and gentle client may suddenly turn aggressive.

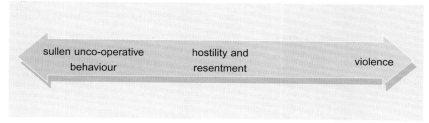

Degrees of aggression

Abuse As discussed in the section on discrimination, abuse is generally either verbal or physical. Once again, some individuals cannot help themselves and express continual, meaningless verbal abuse and use offensive language. Others use it to express themselves because they have learnt no better way of communicating. Clients, however, sometimes abuse their carers as a way of expressing dissatisfaction with a situation.

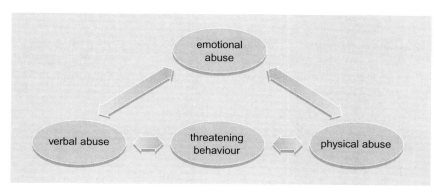

Some types of abuse

Remember that all humans feel the same emotions in different ways. Carers and clients are equally capable of emotional abuse. Think about these situations

- a domineering client ridiculing a less dominant carer

- an aggressive client verbally abusing a carer who is passive

- a carer ridiculing a confused client

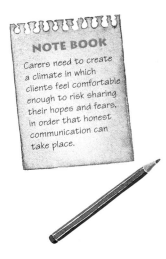

NOTE BOOK

Carers need to create a climate in which clients feel comfortable enough to risk sharing their hopes and fears, in order that honest communication can take place.

ACTIVITY 8

Describe possible positive and negative responses to the following situations.

1 A previously independent older person going into residential care.

2 A parent whose child is diagnosed as having diabetes.

3 Someone with a mental illness being admitted to hospital.

4 A young person with learning difficulties moving into a hostel.

5 Home care services being arranged for a client who is visually impaired.

Record your conclusions imaginatively.

unit four

217

- a carer hitting a client who is weak

- a mentally alert client mocking another who is confused

- an experienced carer being sarcastic to a new member of staff.

All the above situations reflect dissatisfaction and uncertainty in the abuser, however much the opposite may seem to be true. The cause of abuse always needs addressing, whether it is new or established.

Performance Criterion 3

How Different Types of Support May Affect Inter-Personal Relationships Between Clients and Carers

In health and social care work there are various types of support made available to clients. Each type results in a different sort of relationship being formed, depending on the professional role of the carer and the needs of the client. Types of support include information, social, financial, physical, and emotional.

Information

The term **'preventive medicine'** means education in how to avoid becoming ill. It involves the passing on of information about healthy lifestyles, and is as important in terms of saving the country money which would be spent on caring for the sick, as it is promoting personal health and well-being.

In social care, the public needs information on how **benefits** are distributed and who is eligible for them, where advice might be sought, or where practical help comes from.

Information	
Possible client needs	**Carers' attributes**
• information allowing informed choices	• up-to-date, accurate information
• help in deciding what is needed	• effective communication skills
• physical access to information	• may have to travel about to meet client groups.

Social	
Possible client needs	**Carers' attributes**
• to be seen as a guest or friend	• to act as a host or friend
• may have specific care requirements	• may need specific skills to meet client needs
• to develop inter-personal skills	• may have to encourage the development of inter personal skills.
• may need mental / physical / emotional therapy	• may need to deliver mental / physical / emotional therapy.

Social support (day centres, clubs, recreation)

Social support may be provided by day centres, clubs, recreation facilities.

As social animals, people need to meet and communicate with others. Loneliness is bad for physical, mental and emotional health, and can become a habit which individuals may not feel strong enough to break. Social occasions provide opportunities for people to meet one another. It cannot always be assumed that those with a similar complaint will like one another, so clients need a selection of options.

Voluntary services and community groups often provide clubs and day centres. The private sector may do the same, but in a smaller way, some residential care homes offer day care facilities to local informal carers.

Financial support

Help with money matters often begins with an information-gathering process. If a client's financial state has to be explored, this needs to be carried out in a sensitive manner, while at the same time making sure that accurate details are obtained.

Then the distribution of funds takes over. Claims are usually made on paper. Some clients will need help filling in forms or understanding for which benefits they are eligible. A carer may need to do this for them, or explain the process clearly. This could be the role of a key worker, community care worker, or informal carer. The client may be unable to read, not understand English, or be visually impaired.

Physical support

When clients are admitted to hospital, everything is automatically provided. When they are looked after in the community, they need access to all the things they might require to make the most of their independence and make their lives as pleasant as possible. This applies to their families too.

Equipment is provided by the local authority or loaned from the Red Cross and provision varies according to the locality. The local authority will adapt homes to be safer both inside and outside, for example by providing ramps and stair lifts. Local authorities also provide home helps to give assistance with daily living tasks and domestic work. Payment may be according to income. A patient under the care of a community nurse may have continence pads and other aids provided free or on prescription. Again, this varies from district to district. The National Health Service funds nurses and health care workers to make domiciliary (that is, home) visits for nursing and personal care, such as washing, toileting, giving medicines and renewing dressings.

Financial

Possible client needs

- sensitive exploration of financial situation
- help in negotiating paperwork
- review that entitlements are being provided.

Carers' attributes

- sensitivity to clients' feelings
- understanding paperwork
- knowledge of client rights to benefits and exemptions.

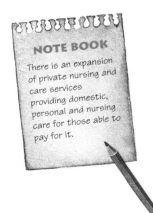

NOTE BOOK

There is an expansion of private nursing and care services providing domestic, personal and nursing care for those able to pay for it.

unit four

219

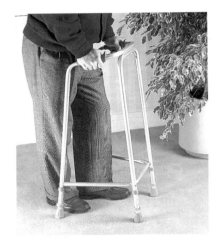
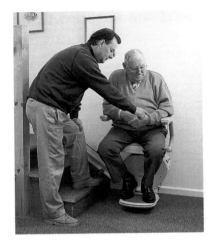
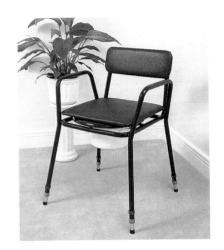

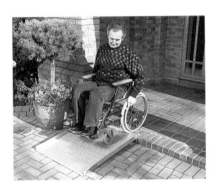
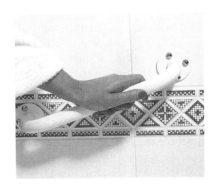
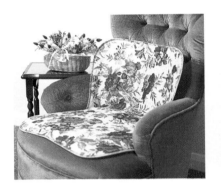

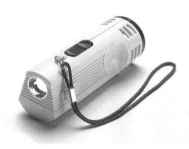
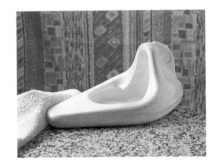
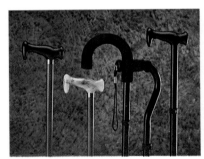

Physical

Possible client needs

1 knowledge of what resources are available locally.
2 home adaptations
3 Home Help
4 personal help and care.

Carers involved

1 key worker, health care worker, social worker, heath visitor, Citizens Advice Bureau, GP, district nurse
2 and 3 as 1 above, then from social services department of local authority
4 community nursing team, private sector carers, community care team.

Emotional support

The large, unpaid army of informal carers looking after relatives at home have many demands made of them, not the least of which are emotional ones. Professional carers come and go off duty, or hand over to a colleague. When client and carer are with one another day in and day out, they may not be able to judge the situation clearly.

Day care gives client and carer a break from one another, to recharge their batteries and gather emotional strength. **Respite care** means day and night spells in hospital, hospice or residential care, either while the carer has a holiday or to provide a change. Respite care is provided by state or private agencies, and sometimes by voluntary support groups.

We are all used to the concept of baby-sitting, but some families need granny/grandad sitting or son/daughter sitting so that the carer can pursue some outside interest.

Children as carers are a small but growing group, as it becomes socially acceptable for adults with disabilities to marry and have children. Or a brother or sister as young as ten years of age may help a working parent with a sibling with a disability. Such carers may be invisible to the support services and unable to discover any help to which they are entitled.

The diagram below summarises the client/carer relationship in terms of emotional support.

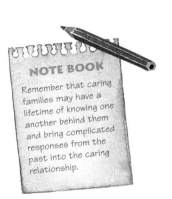

NOTE BOOK

Remember that caring families may have a lifetime of knowing one another behind them and bring complicated responses from the past into the caring relationship.

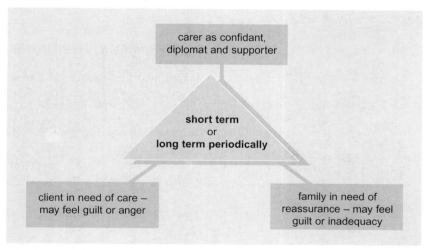

Client/carer relationship – emotional support

Performance Criterion 4

The Role of Effective Interaction in Caring Relationships

When inter-personal communication between client and carer is effective, then something positive emerges. The positive aspects examined here are client empowerment, acknowledgement of personal beliefs and identity, building self-esteem, and building self-confidence.

unit four

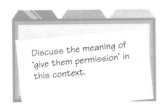

Discuss the meaning of 'give them permission' in this context.

Client empowerment

When someone is empowered, they are given strength, which means emotional strength rather than physical power. The balance of power in the client/carer relationship was examined in pc 1 of this element. Now we are to explore how a carer can give a client power of his or her own. Because of traditional views of patients and others who need looking after, clients often fall into an expected role of dependence, and it can be quite difficult to 'give them permission' to exercise power of their own.

It is achieved by

- letting them know this is acceptable
- encouraging independence
- giving access to choices
- education in lifeskills as well as traditional subjects
- maximising communication skills
- getting to know clients as individuals and allowing them to be themselves
- helping them to behave as accepted members of society.

Acknowledgement of personal beliefs and identity

Before clients can develop their own beliefs they need access to ideas and concepts, and help in understanding them.

With many this takes place during their childhood, and their beliefs may be firmly established before they are in need of care. For those who are 'clients' from infancy, or who may be brought up in institutions, it is part of the caring role to provide opportunities for spiritual enrichment and discussion of abstract opinions within the client's abilities. In this way people discover who they are.

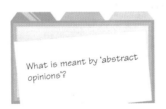

What is meant by 'abstract opinions'?

If individuals are given stereotyping labels their identity is lost and they cease to be seen as themselves. It works both ways, that is both client and carer are often stereotyped. No one likes to be perceived merely as a role.

Carer and client need to see one another as individuals and accept each other's beliefs, whether or not they are shared.

Building self-esteem

Self-esteem means how you value yourself. Confident people feel good about themselves and have high self-esteem. People who see themselves as having no value have low self-esteem. The table below compares the attributes of people with high and low self-esteem.

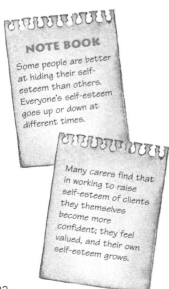

NOTE BOOK

Some people are better at hiding their self-esteem than others. Everyone's self-esteem goes up or down at different times.

Many carers find that in working to raise self-esteem of clients they themselves become more confident; they feel valued, and their own self-esteem grows.

Self-esteem matters for carers as well as clients. Its foundations are laid in childhood, so carers working with children need to be aware of its importance.

Self-esteem

People with high self-esteem
have a realistic view of their abilities, even if they are few
have confidence
are not worried by criticism
enjoy well being
join in willingly
make friends easily
succeed
are independent

People with low self-esteem
underestimate what they can do
are inward looking and unconfident
are sensitive to criticism
get depressed easily
join in reluctantly
find it hard to make friends
underachieve
find independence difficult

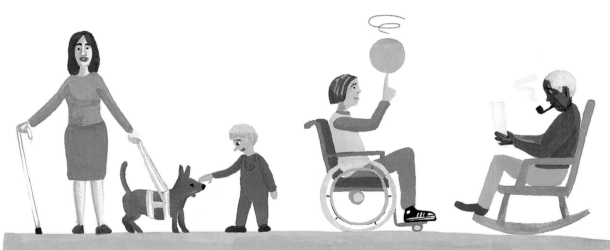

Clients' self-esteem is raised by
- praise
- encouragement
- the chance to make decisions
- being listened to

- independence
- feeling valued
- the chance to succeed
- belonging to a group

- having responsibility
- having even small efforts acknowledged

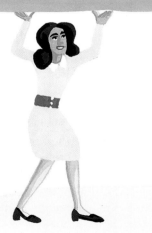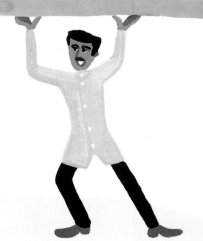

Self-esteem

unit four

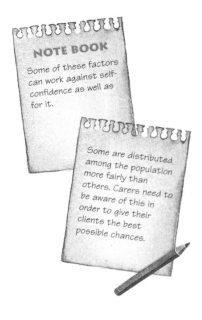

NOTE BOOK

Some of these factors can work against self-confidence as well as for it.

Some are distributed among the population more fairly than others. Carers need to be aware of this in order to give their clients the best possible chances.

Building self-confidence

Empowerment + a feeling of identity + high self-esteem = self confidence. This literally means being confident in one's self rather than relying on others. The media tells us of many individuals who appear to be overwhelmingly handicapped by illness, misfortune or disability, who nevertheless run in marathons, write books, achieve awards and pursue fulfilling careers against all the odds.

This shows that with certain advantages everyone can grow into a self-reliant person, capable of operating independently within their abilities. They sometimes achieve beyond anyone's expectations..

The factors contributing to the self-confidence of individuals are

- personality
- family
- quality of care
- dedication of carers
- support from the state
- effective treatment
- equality of access
- funds
- locality.

Performance Criterion 5

Why Confidentiality is of Critical Importance in Health and Social Care Settings

Confidentiality has a key role to play in client rights, client choices, and building trust. It is important to realise that there can be no such thing as **absolute confidentiality**; this is discussed in pc 6.

Client rights

Clients have equal rights with all citizens, which includes their rights to **privacy**, their own idea of **sexuality** and **personal beliefs**.

They have a right to **information** about legal matters, grievance and complaints systems, and the need for their consent to certain treatments and procedures. This may involve the appointment of an advocate. (See Element 3.2.) Formal care settings have established procedures to protect rights which need to be understood equally by carers and their clients.

Client choices

Clients may need to be encouraged to say what they would prefer. Those who would be confused by too much may need to be offered **guided choice**. This means that the choice is made less confusing by someone else first choosing a small number of equally suitable options. It is important that all workers in the establishment understand this and that it is explained to the client in a way which can be understood.

Choice includes matters of

- food

- clothing

- leisure activities

- independence.

Sometimes clients may make unwise choices which could put them or others at risk, or which would interfere with other people's rights. If this occurs it must be explained in a way which can be understood by those concerned. In the same way, clients' rights to choices have to be observed against the background of the care setting. Sometimes this limits the amount of choice available to clients.

Building trust

Often the carers delivering the most intimate care for clients, such as toileting and bathing, are those who may be regarded as being in the lowliest areas of work. These include care assistants, classroom assistants, and health care workers. Yet they are in a privileged position, as they receive many of the most personal and private confidences of clients. A close relationship is thus built, with the client placing great trust in the carer. Carers in administrative or senior positions may have moved away from this special friendship, and they may rely on junior staff to discover aspects of clients' lives and personalities which are not directly concerned with treatment and care.

Clients need to know that their carers will treat any information they are given as confidential.

In order to do this

- records containing client's details are kept securely according to the establishment's procedures

- written records should not contain explicit or unnecessary detail

- confidential information should be passed on in a suitably private environment

- anything of a personal nature relating to clients is never discussed outside the workplace.

unit four

Performance Criterion 6

The Ethical Issues Which Individuals May Face in Relation to Maintaining Confidentiality

A further complexity in the relationship between client and carer is that of the **ethical nature** of the work. The health and social care services have commitment to personal care and self-advocacy. They have deeply rooted ethical values to consider, if clients are not to be placed at a disadvantage, exploited or damaged during the caring process.

It is difficult for any carer to promise full confidentiality to a client.

Here we will be examining over-riding confidentiality, disclosing information, and the balance between client rights and those of others.

Over-riding confidentiality

Carers have a dilemma if they learn something about a client which they think should be told to senior staff, while feeling a loyalty to the person in their care. The following reference points may help to clarify the situation.

1 Clients must be told in a way they can understand that sometimes personal information must be shared.

2 Such information is only given to those who need and have a right to know about it.

3 If confidential information reveals that anyone will be put at risk, it must be passed on. This could include

- information about drugs/medication being taken without the care team's knowledge

- client plans to damage his or her own or other people's health or well-being

- personal information about past or present behaviour which may affect the client's treatment.

Disclosing information

Usually friends and family are involved when a client needs care. This widens the range of responsibility for carers who have to consider their professional duty to

- management

- colleagues

- clients

- client's friends and family

- the public.

There may be times when the client is being coerced by those outside the care team for information about treatment, domestic details, or maybe legal matters.

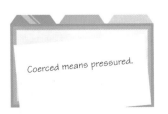

Coerced means pressured.

The same may happen for the carer, and it may be hard to decide how much or how little information to share.

- Carers should not give personal information about clients to other people until this has been discussed with line managers.
- Clients should be protected against stressful pressure from others by their carers. Again, guidance should be sought from senior staff.
- Carers should not agree to act as witnesses for clients or their relatives or friends unless this has been expressly approved by senior management, and certainly never if they are below the age of 18.

The balance between client's rights and those of others

A client's well-being has always to be considered within the context of the organisation which is providing the care. Everybody else has to be thought of at the same time. This means:

- other clients

- their family and friends

- care staff

- others connected with that client's care plan.

ACTIVITY 9

Discuss and record possible conflict of rights in the situation below.

- In residential care, other people's routines may dictate that eccentric time keeping has to be discouraged.
- Loud music is considered inconsiderate when it disturbs others.
- Pregnant women may prefer not to have a male midwife.
- An able-bodied caving society feels unable to cater for the needs of a visually-impaired student who wants to participate.
- An Asian women speaking very little English applies to work in a residential setting with young people with communication difficulties.

unit four

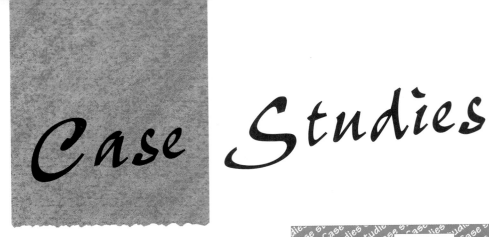

Case Studies

Case study 1   The Thatched Cottage

When Gertrude was first admitted to residential care, she appeared to be a grumpy, aggressive old lady. She complained that her eyes hurt when her curtains were drawn back, hoarded food in her wardrobe, and refused to speak to her relatives when they visited. They needed to discuss her finances with her, but she turned off her hearing aid and went and sat in the bathroom with the door shut. Mark was amazed to hear that she had once been like this, as three months later he knows her as a lively, kind and outgoing person.

Task 1

1 What responses to needing care could Gertrude have been exhibiting when she first joined the Thatched Cottage?

2 What effective interaction might the staff have used to help her to settle?

Task 1

3 Which different types of support might have been given to make life easier for Gertrude and her relatives?

Task 2

1 Work out Isabel's relationships
   a with her family
   b within the school.

   What groups of people is she likely to mix with in each role?

Case study 2   Down Way School

It is a hot day, all the children are too hot to get up to mischief over lunch, and in the shade of the sycamore tree, Isabel is talking to Jalwinder about her work. Jalwinder asks how having had her own children has helped Isabel to be a good classroom assistant. Isabel says that it has been very useful, but that the roles are quite different even though they support one another. Then she has a little doze, and Jalwinder does a bit of thinking while she looks up into the branches of the tree. She doesn't particularly want to have a family, but she does want to stay working with children.

Task 2

2 If Jalwinder remains in child care work and sticks to her resolution not to have a family, how might her relationships within her job be different from Isabel's with her family in terms of
   • dependence

Task 2

   • self management
   • perceived equality of relationships, power, knowledge and understanding.

3 Relate your answer in both cases to the groups of people you have identified in step 1.

Case study 3   Netherfield Community Care

It has been a bad day at the Community Care office. One of the clients with clinical depression has tried to commit suicide, and the team is having a meeting to discuss future management of her case. Debbie is included, as she had reported to Mikhail the week before that this client had told her in confidence that she intended to take her own life. The client had become distressed when Debbie had stated that she would have to report the information, and Debbie feels guilty that she may have contributed to the client's action.

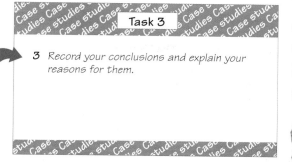

Task 3

1 Discuss whether or not Debbie was justified in reporting the client's confidences to Mikhail.

2 Why is confidentiality so important in health and social care setting?

Task 3

3 Record your conclusions and explain your reasons for them.

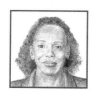

Case study 4   Hill Hall

Ann is impressed by Molly's professionalism. She always seems to know exactly how to respond, even in unexpected circumstances. One day a relative of one of the children asks very persistently for information about treatment and the child's possible progress. Molly is very cool and business-like in her response. When they discuss this over coffee one day, Molly is a bit off-hand, and says 'It's dead easy; you just have to think of them all as special people, and realise at the same time that we all have to get on together here.' Ann mentions this in class when she gets back to college, and they discuss the ethical issues involved.

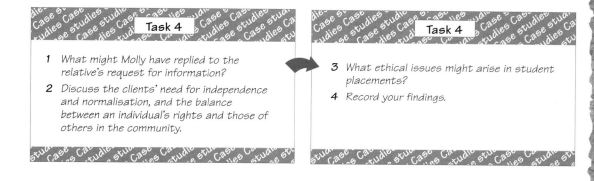

Task 4

1 What might Molly have replied to the relative's request for information?

2 Discuss the clients' need for independence and normalisation, and the balance between an individual's rights and those of others in the community.

Task 4

3 What ethical issues might arise in student placements?

4 Record your findings.

unit four **case studies**

Multiple Choice Questions

1 Balancing clients' rights with those of others is an issue of

   a ethics

   b confidentiality

   c ethics

   d acknowledgement

2 Which of the following is a negative response to receiving care?

   a relief

   b withdrawal

   c reduced stress

   d reduced distress

3 Which statement best describes the importance of confidentiality?

   a it respects clients' rights and builds trust

   b it gives clients physical support in the community

   c it is one of the differences between formal and informal care

   d it is part of the dependence of clients and carers

4 Which type of support is offered by respite care?

   a information and social

   b social and financial

   c financial and physical

   d physical and emotional

5 Effective interaction in caring means

   a providing support for clients

   b helping clients to become dependent

   c undertaking daily living tasks for clients

   d empowering the client

6 Which of the following is a valid reason for telling a client that confidentiality cannot be guaranteed?

   a when the client responds aggressively

   b to acknowledge the client's identity

   c when the caring relationship is at risk

   d when the carer is uncertain of his/her ability to respond effectively

Note: These questions are for you to test your knowledge. There is no formal multiple choice test for Unit 4.

Summary of Evidence Opportunities and Their Relationship to Performance Criteria

Activities 1–6	pc 1	Case study 1	pcs 2, 3 and 4
Activities 7 and 8	pc 2	Case study 2	pcs 1 and 4
Activity 9	pc 6	Case study 3 and 4	pc 5

Unit 4 Element 3 Summary of Element Range and Personal Evidence Tracking Record

Element range references *(tick against left-hand column)*	Description of evidence	Pc and range covered	Portfolio reference number
Pc 1 The caring relationship			
dependence of clients and carers			
extent to which clients can be self-managing			
perceived equality of relationship			
perceived power			
perceived knowledge and understanding of the situation			
Pc 2 Client responses			
positive			
negative			
Pc 3 Types of support			
information			
social			
financial			
physical			
emotional			
Pc 4 The role of effective interaction			
client empowerment			
acknowledgement of personal beliefs and identity			
building self-esteem			
building self-confidence			
Pc 5 Confidentiality			
client rights			
client choice			
building trust			
Pc 6 Ethical issues			
over-riding confidentiality			
disclosing information			
balancing clients rights with those of others			

unit four

As the GNVQ standards are closely followed in the text, words included in them can also be found through the Contents page and the performance criteria page references at the beginning of each element.

access to services **150-151**
advocacy **153**
Aids 21
airway **62**
alcohol 21, 23, 124
balance **19-22**
behaviour 115-116, 181, 216
benefits 135, 148
bleeding (see also haemorrhage) 67
body language **177**, 198
breathing (see also respiration) 39, **61**, **64**
calcium **23**
carbohydrate **22**, 25
cardio pulmonary resuscitation - CPR **64**
career routes **164**
casualty 57-67
celibacy 21
change **100**
choice **124**, 174, 222, 224
circulation 38, 58, **59-60**, 65
classification **119-124**
client groups **145**, 148, 163
Commission for Racial Equality **204**
communication skills **173**, **185**, 222
confidentiality 152, 196, **224**
culture 84, **87**, 98, 117, 152, **195**
day care 219
drug dependency **26-27**
diet **22-25**, 37, 38
dignity 28, **58**, 212
discrimination **193-205**
divorce **106**
drug abuse **26-27**
emergencies **57-67**, 135, 151
emotional support **221**
empowerment 80, **222**
environment
    in development 75
    safe **51-56**
    social **122**
Equal Opportunities Commission **204**, 205
Equal Pay Act **205**
equality **203-205**, 212
ethnicity **195**
evaluation 45, 185
exercise **20**, 36
eye contact **177**, 198
Fair Employment Act **205**
fat **21-22**, 25
feedback 45, 185

fibre **24**, 25
fitness levels **38-40**
funding 131, 133, **135**
gender 85, 194, 203
group settings 113
haemorrhage **67**
hazards **51-56**
health and safety **29**, **51-56**, 118
hearing 28, 80, 146, 179, 183
homelessness **107**
housing **122**, 148
hygiene
    food **29**
    personal **28**
    treatment areas **29**
income 123, 124
independence 75, **81**, 104, 201, 219, 225
independent sector **133**
infection 29, 52, 182
informal care **134**, 136, **162**, 221
interaction **113**, 176, 221
iron **23**
key worker 219, 220
learning difficulties/disabilities 81, 85, **147**, 153, 174, 181
legislation **203**
life saving techniques **62-67**
life stages **74**
lifestyle **19**, 36, 87, 218
listening 80, 173, 177, **179**
mental illness 28, 106, 135, 217
minerals **23**
non-verbal communication 181, 183
normalisation **82**, 181
obesity 39
observation 75, **181**
obstacles to communication **182**
plan **41-42**
primary care **130**
priorities 41
privacy 28, **58**, 224
private sector **133**, 136, 161, 162
provider **131**, **132**, 136
pulse **38-39**, **59**, 65, 67
purchaser **131**, **132**
questions 45, **179**
race **195**, 198
Race Relations Act 203, **204**
racial discrimination **198**, 203, 204
recovery position **63-64**

referral **150-151**
relationships 82, 84, 87, **100-104**, 200, 210, 218
residential care 132, 133, 136
respiration **61**
respite care 162, **221**
responding skills **177**
response 81, **90**, **215-216**
resuscitation **59**, 61, **64-66**
rights 151, 198, **203**, **224**, 227
risk 51
risks to health 41
role 85, 101, **104-105**, **113-119**, 166
safety 20, **51-56**
secondary care **130**
self-advocacy 226
self-concept **84**, 101
self-confidence **224**
self-esteem 75, 105, 201, **222-223**
Sex Discrimination Acts **203**, 205
sexual behaviour 21, 85
sexually transmitted disease 21
shock 58
smoking 21, 90, 124
social classification **119-121**
social services **130-133**, 135, 138, 150, 161, 204
society 104, **113**, 117-119, 222
special needs (see also learning difficulties) **147**, 148
standard measures of health **38-40**
statutory services **130-133**
stereotypes 85, 116, 166, **199**
substance abuse **26-27**
support 58, 91
    by family **105**
    support groups 134, 136
    for client groups **151-153**
support services **159-162**
target groups **43**
tertiary care **130**
touch 81, 146, 177, **179**, 196
unconsciousness **62**
unemployment 119
visual impairment 146
vitamins **23**, 25
voluntary organisations 91, **133**, 136
withdrawal **216**

Buckinghamshire College Group
Wycombe Campus